A Selection Of Words Of Wisdom And Affirmations For Meaningful Living And Happiness

Prof. Alexander D. Wozuzu. Acholonu
PhD, FNSP, FRAES, FMAS, FAS, OON,
Emeritus Professor of Biology
Alcorn State University
Lorman, MS, USA

Copyright by Prof. Alexander D. Wozuzu Acholonu 2023

Printed, 2023
By Advance Publications

Queens, New York 11423

All rights reserved

ISBN: 978-1-951670-57-3 (Paperback)
ISBN: 978-1-951670-58-0 (Digital)

No part of this book may be reproduced or transmitted, downloaded, reverse engineered, or stored in or introduced into any information storage and retrieval system in any form or by any means, including photocopy and recording, whether electronic or mechanical, now known or hereinafter invented, without permission in writing from the publisher.

Printed in the United States of America.

A Selection Of Words Of Wisdom And Affirmations For Meaningful Living And Happiness

Prof. Alexander D. Wozuzu. Acholonu
PhD, FNSP, FRAES, FMAS, FAS, OON,
Emeritus Professor of Biology
Alcorn State University
Lorman, MS, USA

DEDICATION

This book is dedicated, with love, to my seven children who showed unusual fatherly love to and for me both by words and actions:

Anderson Akopoazu
Sandra Akunna
Cynthia Onyemauchechukwu
Leslie Onyemaechi
Esther Eberegbulam
Alexandra Kaonyeuyoaso
Alexander Jr, Dozienze and
The memory of my wife, Lolo, Lady
Mary Ekeoma Acholonu

PS: These are the English and Igbo names I gave them.

Contents

DEDICATION IV
FOREWORD XVI
PREFACE XIX
ACKNOWLEDGEMENTS XXII
SOME DEFINITIONS XXIV

A 1
    Ability 2
    Accomplishment 3
    Achievement 4
    Action 7
    Activity 9
    Adaptability 10
    Adversity 10
    Advice 12
    Affirmations 14
    Ageing 15
    Agreement 15
    Alcoholism 17
    Ambition 17
    Anger 19
    Appearance 21
    Appreciation 22
    Arguments 24
    Asking 26
    Aspiration 26
    Attention 27

Attitude	28
Authority	30

B 31

Balance	32
Baldness	32
Beauty	33
Behavior	33
Belief	36
Benevolence	37
Blessings	37
Borrowing	38
Bosses	39
Brain	40
Business	41

C 43

Carefulness	44
Caution	44
Change	45
Character	47
Charity	49
Choice	50
Circumstances	51
Commitment	52
Commonsense	53
Community	53
Compassion	54
Complaint	55
Compliments	56
Compromise	56
Conceit	57
Condemnation	59
Confidence	59

Confrontation 62
Conscience 62
Consistency 64
Contentment.. 65
Control 66
Contrition 67
Conversation 68
Conviction 69
Cooperation 70
Correction 71
Counseling 71
Courage 72
Crime... 74
Criticism 75
Curiosity 78

D... 79
Death 80
Debts 81
Deeds 83
Defeat 83
Destiny 84
Determination... 84
Dexterity 85
Difficulties... 86
Dignity.. 88
Diplomacy 88
Direction... 89
Disagreement 90
Discipline.. 90
Doubt 92
Dreams.. 92
Duty 93

E 95

- Economy 96
- Education 97
- Ego 99
- Encouragement 101
- Endurance 102
- Enemies 102
- Enjoyment 104
- Enthusiasm 105
- Envy 106
- Equality 107
- Evil 108
- Excellence 109
- Excesses 109
- Excuses 110
- Exercise 111
- Expectations 113
- Experience 113
- Experts 115
- Extravagance 116

F 117

- Facts 118
- Failure 119
- Faith 121
- Fame 124
- Family 124
- Faults 125
- Fear 127
- Feelings 129
- Fight 129
- Finance 130
- Flattery 131
- Focus 131

>   Food 132
>   Foolishness 133
>   Forgiveness 133
>   Fortune 136
>   Frankness 136
>   Freedom 137
>   Friends 138
>   Friendship 140
>   Fruits 142
>   Future 143
>
> G 145
>   Genealogies 146
>   Generosity 146
>   Genius 148
>   Gentleness 149
>   Gifts 149
>   Giving 150
>   Goals 152
>   Godliness 153
>   Goodness 155
>   Grace 156
>   Gratitude 157
>   Greatness 158
>   Growth 160
>   Guidance 161
>
> H 162
>   Habits 163
>   Happiness 163
>   Harmony 165
>   Hatred 166
>   Healing 167
>   Health 168

Heart	169
Help	171
Helpfulness	172
History	172
Hoarding	173
Home	174
Honesty	175
Honor	177
Hope	177
Humanity	179
Humility	181
Humor	183
Hypocrisy	184
I	**185**
Idleness	186
Ignorance	187
Imagination	189
Importance	190
Improvement	191
Independence	192
Industry	192
Inferiority	193
Influence	194
Ingenuity	194
Initiative	195
Insatiability	196
Inscription	196
Insistence	197
Inspiration	197
Instructions	198
Intelligence	198
Intentions	199
Interaction	200

Interest 200
Invention 201
Irresponsibility 201

J 203
Jealousy 204
Journey 204
Joy 205
Judgement 206
Justice 207

K 208
Kindness 209
Knowledge 211

L 214
Lateness 215
Laughter 215
Laziness 216
Leaders 217
Learning 218
Liberty 218
Life 219
Listening 221
Living 222
Loneliness 223
Love 224
Loyalty 226
Luck 227
Lying 228

M 229
Marriage 230
Memory 232
Mind 233
Mistakes 235

Modesty	237
Money	238
Mothers	240
Mutualism	240
N	**242**
Nature	243
Needs	243
O	**245**
Obesity	246
OBSTACLE	246
Offerings	247
Opinions	248
Opportunity	249
Optimists	251
P	**254**
Parenthood	255
Partnership	255
Patience	256
Patriotism	258
Peace	259
Persistence	260
Perfection	261
Perseverance	262
Pessimists	264
Plan	265
Pleasure	266
Politics	267
Popularity	268
Poverty	269
Power	270
Praise	272
Prayer	273

  Prejudice 274
  Prevention 275
  Pride 276
  Principles 276
  Procrastination 277
  Proficiency 279
  Progress 280
  Promises 281
  Prosperity 282
  Protection 283
  Prudence 284

Q 285
  Questioning 286

R 287
  Relationship 288
  Reliability 289
  Repentance 290
  Reputation 290
  Resentment 292
  Respect 292
  Responsibility 293
  Revenge 294
  Riches 295
  Righteousness 296
  Risk 297
  Rumors 297

S 299
  Sacrifice 300
  Safety 300
  Satisfaction 300
  Sayings 302
  Secrets 303

Self-Control 304
Self-Love 306
Selfishness 307
Self-Worth 308
Service 309
Sight 309
Silence 310
Sincerity 312
Solitude 314
Speech 314
Spouse 315
Steadfastness 317
Stinginess 317
Strength 318
Success 320
Suspicion 322
Sympathy 322

T 325
Tact 326
Teaching 327
Temper 328
Temptation 330
Testimony 330
Thankfulness 331
Thoughts 331
Treasure 333
Treatment 333
Thrift 334
Trouble 335
Time 336
Tolerance 336
Trust 337
Truth 338

U	**341**
Understanding	342
Unity	342
Unique	343
V	**344**
Values	345
Verbosity	346
Vices	347
Victory	347
Virtue	348
Vision	349
Vocation	350
W	**352**
War	353
Weakness	353
Wealth	354
Wickedness	355
Will	355
Wisdom	356
Words	358
Worth	360
Work	361
Worry	363
Z	**366**
Zeal	367
PRAYER/SONG AFFIRMATIONS	**368**
REFERENCES	**373**
ABOUT THE AUTHOR	**374**

FOREWORD

It is said that art reveals what words conceal. The book you now hold in your hand is truly a work of art and an exquisite masterpiece. Indeed, the words in this book reveal much about how to live, love, laugh, learn, and leave a lasting legacy. The artistic expressions of this work show something far more penetrating: Specifically, the depth and breadth, as well as scope and sequence of these nuggets of knowledge, evince the fact that Chief Acholonu has spent many years, decades, amassing and amalgamating this treasure trove of timeless thought. In reading the book, I garnered this revelation: much as the author has shaped the arrangement, placement, and engagement of these provocative proverbs and prose, he, too, has been greatly shaped by them as well. One need only spend a brief moment with "The Chief" for a timely, thoughtful, and treasurable truth to tumble out. As a beneficiary and collector who has been the beneficiary of conversations at the feet of this Solomonic sage, I have heard many mantras and assimilated not a small few of them as life, learning, and lessons. Let me bless and bequeath you with one such quote that the Chief has blessed and bequeathed to me. Listen to this gem: "Speak less and less. Listen more and more. " This quote is the basis of my recent book, I Want to Hear You: 22 Tips for Artful Listening before, during, and after a Conversation. I am ever grateful that he gave it to me.

With exacting scrutiny, he has brought to bear his scientific genius to the task of putting together adages and aphorisms, prose and proverbs, quotes and quips, sayings and suggestions, wit, and wisdom consistently culled and carefully curated from cultures, countries, and contexts. They are organized for quick reference in alphabetical order. The quotations are satirical, sarcastic, cynical, absurd, frivolous, and exaggerated in some cases. Some are pensive and reflective, while some are for comfort and celebration of meaningful living and the inducement of happiness. The proverbs contain many brief but wise statements, mainly about how to live a godly life.

The book is highly useful for speakers, writers, editors, teachers, and preachers. It contains words of faith and encouragement, lively ideas, commonsense, profound wisdom, and plain good humor for authors of different kinds. The author brought out the fact that his father taught him many proverbs and affirmations and made him memorize them and use them for meaningful, thoughtful, progressive, and godly living. Since he found them useful and used them as his guiding principles, he included them in this book to pass them on like a baton to others for their betterment, which was very thoughtful of him.

The book is written in a style that is easy to follow. The author is an academician and a scientist and yet mustered enough courage to write such a useful book not related to science but human behavior. He ought to be highly praised for this milestone or great accomplishment. He said that he did it as an extracurricular activity and also gave credit to his father for the impetus to write it. It is a gem for people from all walks of life and will encourage good living and happiness, as indicated by the title of the book.

I strongly recommend it, especially to teachers, preachers, speakers, and those who want to wax in wisdom.

Dr. John Igwebuike
Former Interim Provost and Executive
Vice President for Academic Affairs
Alcorn State University, Lorman, MS 39096 USA

Present Address
Dr. John G. Igwebuike
Executive Director
Guanacaste: The lead Listening Society
www.leadlisteninginstitue.com

PREFACE

This book is a wisely selected collection of quotations filled with a myriad of clever and pungent sayings to give impetus and zeal to conversations, speeches, and writings. It is a selection of proverbs, platitudes, affirmations, and wise sayings I got from elderly and learned people, and I copied from different books and publications, as can be seen from the list of references. I spent many years of my life gathering the many entries in this useful and captivating book. These words of wisdom and affirmations are organized for quick reference into alphabetically listed subject headings from "A" to "Z". Some of the quotations are satirical, sarcastic, cynical, absurd, frivolous, and exaggerated. Some are pensive and reflective, while some are for comfort and celebration of meaningful living and the inducement of happiness. Every entry is by itself quotable, making the book one of the most enticing and inviting books of its kind. The proverbs contain many brief but wise statements, mainly about how to live a godly life.

It is highly useful for speakers, writers, editors, teachers, preachers, and anyone who wants a short or brief saying at his or her fingertips or the tip of the tongue. It contains words of faith and encouragement, lively ideas, commonsense, profound wisdom, and plain good humor for authors of different kinds. It is an entertaining and useful book for those who relish humor and those who enjoy provocative insight into everything from the righteous to the ridiculous.

As a young man, my father, Mr. Wilfred W. Acholonu, a court clerk and a councilor, taught me many proverbs and affirmations and made me memorize them as a guide to living a meaningful life. The result is that I still remember many of them. Since I have found them useful and use them as my guiding principles, I have included them in this book to pass them on to others so that the knowledge does not die in me; and believing in the words of Confucius: "Has God given you knowledge? Give it to others for their own betterment; give it to them for your own improvement."

In my elementary school days, we were taught proverbs and made to memorize them. We were exposed to *John Plummer's Book of Proverbs*.

I recall that I formally opened a file where I stored these wise statements and words of wisdom I got from people and my readings in 2002.

This book is written in a style that is easy to follow. The chapters are alphabetical and logically sequenced. The affirmations and proverbs are united with words of wisdom since they appear to have similarities in meaning and let the reader make up his mind about which to call which.

It may boggle the mind that an academician and for that matter, a scientist, decided to write a book that has nothing to do with science. This happens to be my side attraction, one of my extracurricular activities, and an interest acquired or cultivated by my father, especially the affirmations.

Chief Sir. Prof. Alexander Dozie Wozuzu Acholonu, PHD, FNSP, FRAES, FMAS, FAS, OON
Emeritus Professor of Biology
Alcorn State University
Lorman, MS, USA

ACKNOWLEDGEMENTS

This book, A Selection of Words of Wisdom and Affirmations for Meaningful Living and Happiness, is the result of hard work, support and input from various people. As I said about the book, thoughts of writing it started in 2002. Since that time, I have selected several words of wisdom and affirmations from different books and gotten a lot from my father, my friends, and several other sources. I am grateful to God for giving me the impetus, the courage, and the inspiration to start and complete this work. My special thanks go to Dr. John Igwebuike, the former Interim Provost and Vice President for Academic Affairs at Alcorn State University who prepared the FOREWORD for the book. I am grateful to those who reviewed the book, namely Dr. Anne-Marie Obilade, Interim Head and Associate Professor, Department of English Language and Mass Communication, and Dr. Eric Dogini, Associate Professor in the Department of Mass Communications. I am grateful to Dr. Charles Obichere and Prof. Simeon Okpechi, who contributed some of the prayers and songs that are included in this book. I am most grateful to my late wife, Lolo Lady Mary Ekeoma Acholonu, and our children, Anderson Akopoazu Acholonu, Sandra Akunna

Acholonu, Mrs. Cynthia Onyemauechi Acholonu-Grant, Lolo Engr. Mrs. Leslie Onyemauchechukwu Acholonu-Okere, Attorney Mrs. Esther Eberegbulam Acholonu Streete, Mrs. Alexandra Kaonyeuyoaso Acholonu Matthis and Alexander Dozienze Wozuzu Acholonu Jr. for their moral support and various inputs in making this book a reality.

I acknowledge the clerical and technical assistance given to me by my daughter, Mrs. Cynthia Acholonu Grant; my granddaughter, Nnawuhe Sinachi Streete; and my students, Sharkiesha Jackson and Emmanuel Ufio, a Nigerian student at Alcorn State University. They demonstrated interest and exercised admirable patience during the preparation of this book.

Chief Sir. Prof. Alex Dozie Wozuzu Acholonu,
PHD, FNSP, FRAES, FMAS, FAS, OON
Emeritus professor
Alcorn State University.

Some definitions

What is Affirmation?
Answer: "Affirmations in New Thought and New Age terminology refer primarily to the practice of positive thinking and self-empowerment—fostering a belief that "a positive mental attitude supported by affirmations will achieve success in anything." More specifically, an affirmation is a carefully formatted statement that should be repeated to one's self and written down frequently. For affirmation to be effective, it is said that they need to be present tense, positive, personal and specific." – *Oxford English Dictionary*

What are "Words of Wisdom"?
Answer: "Accumulated knowledge or erudition or enlightenment. The trait of utilizing knowledge and experience with commonsense and insight. Ability to apply knowledge or experience and understanding. The quality of being prudent and sensible." – *Wolfram Alpha Words of wisdom means very wise remarks*

What is another word for "Words of Wisdom"?

Answer: Proverb, saying, adage, maxim, aphorism, axiom, dictum, truism, motto. – *WordHippo.com*

What is Wisdom?

"Wisdom is the ability to contemplate and act using knowledge, experience, understanding, common sense and insight" – *Oxford English Dictionary*

"The quality of having experience, knowledge and good judgement; the quality of being wise. The soundness of an action or decision with regard to the application of experience, knowledge and good judgement." – *Oxford Languages Dictionary*

The Symbols and their Meaning

 Nokore — Truth. Symbol of Truth

 Nea Onnim — Nea Onnim means "He who does not know." It is from the Akan proverb, "Nea Onnim no sua a ohu." which translates as, "When he who does not know learns, he gets to know."

 Sesa Wo Suban — Change or transform your Character. Symbol of life transformation.

 Dwennimmen — Dwennimmen means "the horns of a ram." It represents strength (in mind, body, and soul), humility, wisdom, and learning.

Nyansapo — "Wisdom knot"

Symbol of wisdom, ingenuity, intelligence and patience.

An especially revered symbol of the Akan, this symbol conveys the idea that, "a wise person has the capacity to choose the best means to attain a goal. Being wise implies broad knowledge, learning and experience, and the ability to apply such faculties to practical ends."

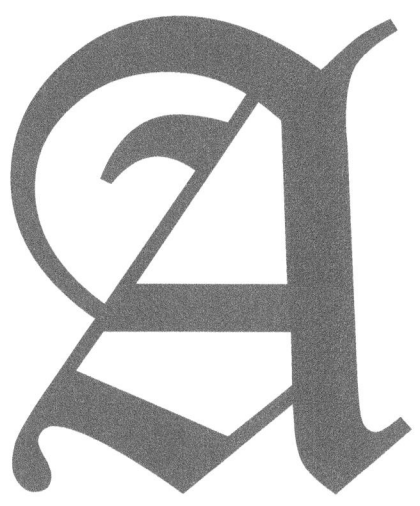

ABILITY

- Ability will enable a man to get to the top, but it takes character to keep him there. – *American Proverb*

- Ability without ambition is like a car without a motor.

- Be big enough to admit and admire the abilities of people who are better than you are.

- Believe you can and you're halfway there. – *Theodore Roosevelt*

- Don't envy anybody. Everyone has something that no one else does. Develop that one thing and make it outstanding.

- It is better to have a little ability and use it well than to have a lot of ability and make poor use of it.

- No man is fully accomplished until he has acquired the ability to attend to his own business.

- The tragedy is that so many have ambition and so few have ability. – *William Feather*

- There is great power in letting go, and there is great freedom in moving on. – *Bruce Van Horn*

- We increase our ability, stability, and responsibility when we increase our sense of accountability to God.

- We rate the ability of men by what they finish, not by what they attempt.

- What lies behind us and what lies before us are tiny matters compared to what lies within us. – *Ralph Waldo Emerson*

- You can do everything you ought to do.

- You cannot run faster than your legs can carry you.

Accomplishment

- I find happiness in helping others to achieve the same.

- I am happy because of my past accomplishments, but I do not dwell on those achievements since I am living in the present.

- Some fellows dream of worthy accomplishments, while others stay awake and do them. – *Ziad K. Abdelnour*

- No man is fully accomplished until he has acquired the ability to attend to his own business.

- As you sow, so shall you reap. – *Galatians 6:7*

- There are four steps to accomplishment: Plan purposefully. Prepare prayerfully. Proceed positively. Pursue persistently. – *William Arthur Ward*

- It's difficult to inspire others to accomplish what you haven't been willing to try. – *Confucius*

- It is not only what you do, but also what you don't do, for which you are accountable. – *Molière*

- Great things are done by a series of small things brought together. – *Vincent Van Gogh*

Achievement

- You can't make a place for yourself under the sun if you keep sitting in the shade of the family tree.

- It is when we forget ourselves that we do things that are most likely to be remembered.

- Every accomplishment, great or small, starts with the right decision, *"I'll try."*

- The only thing ever achieved in life without effort is failure. – *Francis of Assisi*

- You must first be a believer if you want to be an achiever.

- Today's preparation determines tomorrow's achievement.

- Man's maximum achievement often falls short of God's minimum demands.

- Education is not received. It is achieved. – *Albert Einstein*

- Having money and friends is easy. Having friends and no money is an accomplishment.

- Money, achievement, fame, and success are all important, but they are bought too dearly when acquired at the cost of health.

- Hope sees the invisible, feels the intangible, and achieves the impossible. – *Helen Keller*

- Hope is the anchor of the soul, the stimulus to action, and the incentive to achievement.

- Liberty is not a gift of God but a hard-won achievement with the help of God.

- You cannot control the length of your life, but you can control its breadth, depth, and height.

- The difference between ordinary and extraordinary is that little extra. – *Jimmy Johnson*

- Achievement doesn't come from what you do, but from who you are. Your worldly power results from your personal power. Your career is an extension of your personality. – *Marianne Williamson*

- He who rests, rusts. – *German Provers, "We rastet, der rostet"*

- May your focus be not on what you have achieved so far, but on what you have yet to achieve.

- Set your own pace. Some thrive on huge, dramatic change. Some people prefer the slow and steady route. Do what's right for you. – *Julie Morgenstern*

- College professors are not made overnight. They reach the height of their profession by degree.

ACTION

- Action may not always bring happiness; but there is no happiness without action. – *Benjamin Disraeli*

- "Push" will get a person almost everywhere — except through a door marked "pull."

- A man's conscience tells him what he shouldn't do — but it does not keep him from doing it. – *Frank A. Clark*

- A spoken word and a thrown stone cannot be recalled. – *Swedish Proverb*

- Acting without thinking is a lot like shooting without aiming. – *B.C. Forbes*

- Good intentions are no substitute for action; failure usually follows the path of least persistence.

- Well done is better than well said. – *Benjamin Franklin*

- If you cannot do great things, do smart things in a great way. – *Napoleon Hill*

- There are three kinds of people in this world: those who see things happen, those who wonder about what happened, and those who make things happen. – *John Newbern's Law*

- To get what you want, STOP doing what isn't working. – *Earl Warren*

- What happens is not as important as how you react to what happens. – *Ellen Glasgow*

- Do something. Either lead, follow, or get out of the way! – *Thomas Paine*

- Failure always overtakes those who have the power to do so without the will to act.

- Genius is 1 percent inspiration and 99 percent perspiration. – *Thomas Edison*

- If you itch for success, keep on scratching.

- Never judge a man's actions until you know his motives. – *Vikas Swarup*

- Our words may hide our thoughts, but our actions will reveal them.

- The man who gets ahead is the man who does more than is necessary and keeps on doing it.

❦ The one thing worse than a quitter is a man who is afraid to start. – *Suzanne Woods Fisher*

ACTIVITY

❦ I am actively using my muscles and my limbs rather than being immobile.

❦ I am happy when I am as active as possible, running, walking, swimming, exercising not as a chore but as a gift of being strong enough to work.

❦ Staying busy makes me happy.

❦ If you don't move your body, your brain thinks you're dead. Movement of the body will not only clear out the "sludge," but will also give you more energy. Treat your body like a car, keep it tuned up and it will run for a very long time. – *Sylvia Browne*

❦ Pick up the pace of your life. Add a new activity, make a new acquaintance, read a new book, or take a new course. Move outside your everyday mundane existence. Add a new beat and expand your boundaries. – *Tavis Smiley*

Adaptability

- In matters of style, swim with the current; in matters of principle, stand like a rock. – *Thomas Jefferson*

- Change in all things is sweet. – *Aristotle*

- Don't ask for an easier life, ask for a stronger person.

- Accept the challenges, so that you may feel the exhilaration of victory. – *George S. Patton*

Adversity

- Adversity is the only diet that will reduce a fat head. – *David L. Allen*

- We learn some things from prosperity, but we learn many more from adversity.

- He who swells in prosperity will shrink in adversity. – *Charles Caleb Colton*

- Adversity is never pleasant, but sometimes it's possible to learn lessons from it that can be learned in no other way.

- Your character is what you have left when you've lost everything you can lose. – *Evan Esar*

- The difficulties of life are intended to make us better, not bitter. – *Tiny Buddha*

- There are two ways of meeting difficulties: altering the difficulties or altering yourself to meet them. – *Phyllis Bottome*

- Education is an ornament in prosperity and a refuge in adversity. – *Aristotle*

- All men need a faith that will not shrink when washed in the waters of affliction and adversity.

- The friends you make in prosperity are those you lose in adversity.

- A real friend will tell you your faults and follies in times of prosperity and assist you with his hand and heart in times of adversity.

- Prosperity makes friends; adversity tries them. – *Publilius Syrus*

- ❦ Love is a fabric that never fades, no matter how often it is washed in the water of adversity and grief. – *Rober Fulghum*

- ❦ Most people who sit around waiting for their ship to come in often find it a hardship.

- ❦ In times of prosperity, men ask too little of God. In times of adversity, they ask too much.

ADVICE

- ❦ You sometimes profit from the advice you don't take.

- ❦ Successful men follow the same advice they prescribe for others.

- ❦ Too many people are anxious to give you advice when what you really need is help.

- ❦ We might be more eager to accept good advice if it did not continually interfere with our plans.

- ❦ Advice is the only commodity on the market where the supply always exceeds the demand. – *Anupam Kher*

- An intelligent person not only knows how to take advice but also how to reject it.

- No one gives advice with more enthusiasm than an ignorant person.

- Advice is like medicine—the correct dosage works wonders, but an overdose can be dangerous.

- It takes a great man to give sound advice tactfully, but a greater man to accept it graciously. – *Logan Pearsall Smith*

- Most of us find it impossible to take advice from people who need it more than we do.

- We don't mind if someone wants to give us advice; we only object if they insist we take it.

- Advice is that which the wise don't need and fools won't take. – *Benjamin Franklin*

- Most people, when they come to you for advice, want their opinions strengthened, not corrected.

- The best advice you'll get is from someone who made the same mistake himself.

- A good example has twice the value of good advice. — *Kem Wilson*

- Old age is that period when a man is too old to take advice but young enough to give it.

- Get all the advice and instruction you can, so you will be wise the rest of your life. — *Proverbs 19:20*

- Plans go wrong for lack of advice; many advisers bring success. — *Proverbs 15:22*

- Though good advice lies deep within the heart, a person with understanding will draw it out. — *Proverbs 20:5*

- The godly give good advice to their friends; the wicked lead them astray. — *Proverbs 12:26*

AFFIRMATIONS

- Say positive affirmations each morning to open the gates of manifestation. — *Doreen Virtue, Ph.D.*

- Affirmations work because I am reinforcing positive thinking.

- ❦ I will try to find affirmations that stem from other cultures, and I will benefit from those positive thoughts and concepts.

AGEING

- ❦ Know that you are at the perfect age. Each year is special and precious, for you shall only live it once. Be comfortable with growing older. – *Louise L. Hay*

- ❦ None are so old as those who have cultivated enthusiasm. – *Henry David Thoreau*

- ❦ 40 is the old age of youth; 50 is the youth of old age. – *Victor Hugo*

AGREEMENT

- ❦ A "gentleman's agreement" is a deal which neither party cares to put in writing.

- ❦ A divorce is what couples agree on when they can't agree on anything else.

- About the only thing people in every walk of life will agree about is that they are underpaid and overcharged.

- As soon as you observe that everybody agrees with you, you can be sure they don't mean it.

- It's a pretty safe rule that the fellow who always agrees with you is not worth talking to.

- Reasonable men always agree if they understand what they're talking about.

- Take the responsibility to make new agreements with those you love. If an agreement doesn't work, change the agreement and create a new one. Use your imagination to explore the possibilities. – *Don Miguel Ruiz*

- The man who always agrees with you, lies to others also.

- When you hear an opinion and believe it, you make an agreement and it becomes part of your belief system. The only thing that can break this agreement is to make a new one based on truth. Only the truth has the power to set you free. – *Don Miguel Ruiz*

✤ When you say that you agree to a thing in principle, you mean that you do not have the slightest intention of carrying it out. – *Otton von Bismarck*

ALCOHOLISM

✤ Wine produces mockers; alcohol leads to brawls. Those led astray by drink cannot be wise. – *Proverbs 20:1*

✤ Those who love pleasure become poor; those who love wine and luxury will never be rich. – *Proverbs 21:17*

✤ Drink because you are happy, but never because you are miserable. – *G.K. Chesterton*

AMBITION

✤ We rate the ability of men by what they finish, not by what they attempt.

- Some fellows dream of worthy accomplishments, while others stay awake and do them. – *Ziad K. Abdelnour*

- Every accomplishment, great or small, starts with the right decision, *"I'll try."*

- Don't just stand there — do something! – *Albert Mohler*

- Don't sit back and take what comes. Go after what you want. – *John Mason, An Enemy Called Average*

- The fellow who has an abundance of push gets along very well without any pull.

- Ambition never gets anywhere until it forms a partnership with work. – *James Abram Garfield*

- The average man's ambition is to be able to afford what he's spending.

- Watch out for ambition! It can get you into a lot of hard work.

- The tragedy is that so many have ambition and so few have ability. – *William Feather*

- Ambition without determination has no destination.

- The plain fact is that human beings are happy only when they are striving for something worthwhile.

- Most lazy people have about as much initiative as an echo.

- The man with PUSH will pass the man with PULL.

- If you search for good, you will find favor, but if you search for evil, it will find you! – *Proverbs 11:27*

ANGER

- Hot words never result in cool judgement.

- He who has a sharp tongue soon cuts his own throat. – *Confucius*

- To take the wind out of an angry man's sails, stay calm.

- An angry man is seldom reasonable; a reasonable man is seldom angry.

- Anger is a state that starts with madness and ends with regret. – *Imam Ali*

- The best way to get rid of a hothead is to give him the cold shoulder.

- You shouldn't get angry at someone who knows more than you do. After all, it's not his fault.

- When angry, count to ten before speaking. When very angry, count to one hundred and then don't speak. – *Thomas Jefferson*

- Striking while the iron is hot may be all right, but don't strike while the head is hot.

- Have you noticed that a fire department never fights fire with fire?

- The man who cannot be angry at evil usually lacks enthusiasm for good. – *Dr. David Seamands*

- Be strong enough to control your anger instead of letting it control you.

- Anger is a wind that blows out the lamp of the mind. – *Robert Green Ingersoll*

- Anger makes your mouth work faster than your mind.

- The greatest remedy for anger is delay. – *Seneca*

- As a general rule, the angriest person in a controversy is the one who is wrong.

- Forgiveness saves the expense of anger, the high cost of hatred, and waste of energy. – *Hannah More*

- Patience strengthens the spirit, sweetens the temper, stifles anger, subdues pride, and bridles the tongue. – *George Horne*

- A gentle answer deflects anger, but harsh words make tempers flare. – *Proverbs 15:1*

- Form the habit of closing your mouth firmly when angry.

Appearance

- A father is usually more pleased to have his child look like him than to have him act like him.

- The Lord gives us our faces, but we must provide the expression.

- The surest sign that a man is not great is when he strives to *look* great.

- When happiness gets into your system, it is bound to break out on your face. – *Adi Da*

- It is a mistake to trust a man with an honest face. After all, that may be the only honest part of him.

- There's a facelift you can perform yourself that is guaranteed to improve your appearance. It is called a smile.

- The real secret to looking young is being young.

Appreciation

- I remind myself that it is the little things that mean a lot.

- I am happy because of the little things in life that I take the time to appreciate.

- Appreciating the talents I was born with, makes me happy.

- Someone else appreciating me and praising me is very powerful, but appreciating myself is the most potent of all.

- There is always someone who has more than me and someone who has less than me. Being happy is appreciating what I have without comparing myself to others.

- You must speak up to be heard, but sometimes you have to shut up to be appreciated.

- The best way to appreciate your job is to imagine yourself without one.

- Don't forget that appreciation is always appreciated.

- Appreciation is what some other people lack when you do them a favor.

- It is better to appreciate something you have than to have something you can't appreciate.

- Appreciation makes people feel more important than almost anything you can give them.

- A single rose for the living is better than a costly wreath for the grave.

- Happiness will never come to those who fail to appreciate what they already have. – *Gautama Buddha*

Arguments

- One of the sorriest spectacles imaginable is the anger of two people who have gotten into an argument over something that neither of them knows anything about.

- It will do no good to argue if you're in the wrong, and if you're right — you don't need to.

- The more arguments you win, the fewer friends you'll have.

- A word to the wise usually starts an argument.

- An argument produces plenty of heat but not much light.

- It is impossible to defeat an ignorant man in an argument. – *William G. McAdoo*

- You get out of an argument exactly what you put into it: a lot of hot air.

- In an argument, the best weapon to hold is your tongue.

- Discussion is an exchange of knowledge; an argument is an exchange of ignorance. – *Robert Quillen*

- An argument is when two people are trying to get in the last word first.

- People who know the least always argue the most.

- One thing a man learns from an argument with a woman is how to be a good loser.

- When an argument flares up, the wise man quenches it with silence.

- It is a rare thing to win an argument and the other fellow's respect at the same time.

- An argument is like a country road; you never know where it'll lead.

- Being a gentleman is a worthy trait, but it is a great handicap in an argument.

- There's one thing to be said for ignorance — it causes a lot of interesting arguments.

- It is impossible to win an argument with an ignorant man.

ASKING

- ❦ Asking is the beginning of receiving. Through a simple, believing prayer, you can change your future. You can change what happens one minute from now. – *Dr. Bruce Wilkinson*

- ❦ Ask and you shall receive; knock and it shall be opened unto you.

- ❦ Ask not what your country can do for you, but what you can do for your country. – *JFK*

ASPIRATION

- ❦ Some people see things as they are and say why. I see things as they never were and say why not. – *Bernard Shaw*

- ❦ No one can create in your experience, for no one can control where you direct your thoughts. On the path to your happiness, you will discover all you want to be, do, or have. – *Abraham Hicks*

- Reach for the stars, you might hit the clouds. – *Att. Esther Streete, my daughter*

- Never tell me the sky's the limit when there are footprints on the moon. – *Paul Brandt*

- Think BIG. There are unseen forces ready to support your dreams. – *Cheryl Richardson*

- The fears of the wicked will be fulfilled; the hopes of the godly will be granted. – *Proverbs 10:24*

- There is plenty of room at the top because very few people care to travel beyond the average route. – *Nnamdi Azikiwe*

- Surround yourself with people of equal or greater ability, aptitude, and experience. Tap into new talent, and experience greater growth. Not only will you benefit, but those around you will also prosper. – *Tavis Smiley*

ATTENTION

- Pay attention to what a man is, not what he has been.

- ❦ The quickest way to get a lot of individual attention is to make a big mistake.

- ❦ When you do the common things in life in an uncommon way, you will command the attention of the world. – *George Washington Carver*

ATTITUDE

- ❦ Attitude is the foundation and support for everything you do. It's a key element in the process of controlling your destiny. – *Keith D Harrell*

- ❦ I remind myself to be positive and reinforce a joyful attitude.

- ❦ I know that a positive attitude spreads, so I make an effort to reinforce my positive thoughts.

- ❦ A bowl of vegetables with someone you love is better than a steak with someone you hate.

- ❦ Be civil to all, sociable to many, familiar with few, friend to one, enemy to none. Do things without expecting praise from men. Your rewarder and promoter is God!

- An evil company corrupts good manners. – *1 Corinthians 15:33*

- You catch more flies with honey than with vinegar.

- The latitude of a man's attitude is his altitude. – *Agwa wu mma*

- Don't let the attitude of some ungrateful people stop you from doing favors to others because your rewards come from someone greater than US. – *Dr. Idysuyi*

- Empowering beliefs strengthen you. Today, create and focus on three empowering beliefs that contribute to your positive attitude. – *Keith D. Harrell*

- It is your attitude, not your aptitude, that determines your altitude.

- People can alter their lives by altering their attitudes. – *William James*

- Remove the obstacles. Untangle the clutter of hats standing between you and a productive, fulfilling life. – *Julie Morgenstern*

- Begin to see the invisible so that you can do the impossible. Your positive attitude and it was you have to see beneath the surface so that you can accomplish anything you want. – *Keith D. Harrell*

- Surround yourself with positive people and situations and avoid negativity. - *Doreen Virtue, Ph.D.*

- I am changing myself so that I am more positive and happier.

- The tongue can bring death or life; those who love to talk will reap the consequences.

- Where cruelty and lenity play a game, the gentle gamester is always the winner.

AUTHORITY

- Nothing intoxicates some people like a sip of authority.

- If there's anything small, shallow, or ugly about a person, giving him a little authority will bring it out.

- Question authority but raise your hand first. – *Alan M. Dershowitz*

BEAUTY

- Beauty awakens the soul to act. – *Dante Alighiere*

- Beauty is in the beholder's eye. – *Margaret Wolfe Hungerfold*

- She will place a lovely wreath on your head; she will present you with a beautiful crown. – *Proverbs 4:9*

- No beauty shines brighter than that of a good heart. – *Shanina Shaik*

- When you do not know what to tell a pretty woman, you ask her what you do with beauty.

BEHAVIOR

- Think about what others ought to be like, then start being like that yourself.

- To know what is right and not to do it is as bad as doing it wrong.

- The surest way to gain respect is to earn it through your conduct.

- It's nice to be important, but it's more important to be nice.

- Don't be a carbon copy of something. Make your own impressions.

- You can't hold your head up, but be careful to keep your nose at a friendly level.

- You can't hold another fellow down in the ditch unless you stay down there with him.

- Blowing out the other fellow's candle won't make yours shine any brighter.

- A true test of a man's character is not what he does in the light, but what he does in the dark.

- It isn't what you have, but who you are, that makes life worthwhile.

- When you laugh, be sure to laugh at what people do, not at what people are.

- It is easier to hide mistakes than to prevent their consequences.

- A man must be big enough to admit his mistakes, smart enough to profit from them, and strong enough to correct them. – *John C. Maxwell*

- A man who has made a mistake and doesn't correct it is committing another mistake.

- An open mind and a closed mouth make a happy combination.

- A man's conscience, and not his mattress, has most to do with his sleep.

- Some men succeed because of what they know, others because of what they do, and a few because of who they are.

- Will power cannot be furnished by anyone but you.

- You can catch more flies with honey than with vinegar. – *American Proverb*

- It is foolish to belittle one's neighbor; a sensible person keeps quiet.

BELIEF

- Some things have to be believed to be seen. – *Ralph Hodgson*

- To be a great champion, you must believe you are the best. If you're not, pretend you are. – *Muhammad Ali*

- To walk out of God's will is to step into nowhere. – *C.S. Lewis*

- Take a stand for what you believe in.

- I meditate because finding calm within myself makes me happy.

- Find the courage to hold on to your beliefs even if the world around you chooses to believe differently. Have the courage to change those beliefs that no longer fit the person you have become. In doing so, you truly become yourself. – *Daniel Levin*

- So what if someone was born thinner or stronger, lighter or darker than you? Why can't diplomas or compare resumes? What does it matter if they have a place at the head table? You have a place at God's table. – *Max Lucado*

BENEVOLENCE

- Spontaneously engage in acts of benevolence and generosity. – *Leon Nacson*

- I am reaching out to others who are not as fortunate as I am, and it makes me happy to share.

- It makes me happy to do something for someone else because it might bring that person joy.

- Share your gifts with the world.

BLESSINGS

- I go to sleep at night counting my blessings and I look forward to my dreams and the next day's wonder.

- Discover the blessings you already have. – *Cherie Carter-Scott, Ph.D.*

- Treasure your physical being as a vehicle that houses your soul. Once you have the inner way, the outer way will follow. – *Dr. Wayne W, Dyer*

BORROWING

- An acquaintance is a person whom we know well enough to borrow from but not well enough to lend to.

- When a man borrows money from a bank, he pays interest, but when he borrows from a friend, he often loses interest.

- The trouble with a chronic borrower is that he always keeps everything but his word.

- It is a fraud to borrow when you know that you will be unable to repay.

- Friends last longer, the less they are used.

- You can usually tell how close your closest friend is if you ask him for a loan.

- A friend in need is a drain on the pocketbook.

- A lifelong friend is someone you haven't borrowed money from yet.

- It's strange how much better our memories become as soon as a friend borrows money from us.

- If you want to know the value of money, try and borrow it.

- Before borrowing money from a friend, decide what you need more.

- Sympathy is what you give to a man when you don't want to lend him money.

- Time may be money, but it's much easier to persuade a man to give you his time than to lend you his money.

Bosses

- Before arguing with your boss, make absolutely sure you're right, then let the matter drop.

- Nothing makes a man the boss of his house like living alone.

- The worst boss anyone can have is a bad habit.

- A man's best boss is a well-trained conscience.

- The fellow who is fired with enthusiasm for his work is seldom fired by his boss.

- The fellow who knows more than his boss should be careful to conceal it.

- It is generally understood that leisure time is what you have when the boss is on vacation.

- If you do all the work and somebody else gets the credit, he's probably your boss.

Brain

- Age stiffens the joints and thickens some brains.

- Be sure your brain is engaged before putting your mouth in gear.

- Always remember that a man is not rewarded for having brains, but for using them.

- Most folks would benefit themselves and others if they would synchronize their tongues with their brains.

- Brains and beauty are nature's gifts; character is your own achievement.

- Nature abhors a vacuum. When a head lacks brains, nature fills it with conceit.

- If a person has no education, he is forced to use his brain.

- There are more idle brains than idle hands.

- Your brain becomes a mind when it's fortified with knowledge.

Business

- Doing business without advertising is like winging a girl in the dark. You know what you're doing, but she doesn't.

- A "gentleman's agreement" is a deal which neither party cares to put in writing.

- If you want to go far in business, you'll have to stay close to it.

- In the business world, transactions speak louder than words.

- It isn't the business you get that counts, it's the business you hold.

- The business to stay out of is the other fellow's.

- Business will continue to go where it is invited and will remain where it is appreciated.

- Sign on a company bulletin board in Grand Rapids: *"To err is human, to forgive is not company policy."*

- In the language of flowers, the yellow rose means friendship, the red rose means love, and the orchid means business.

- Humor is the lubricating oil of business. It prevents friction and wins good will.

- The trouble with mixing business and pleasure is that pleasure usually comes out on top.

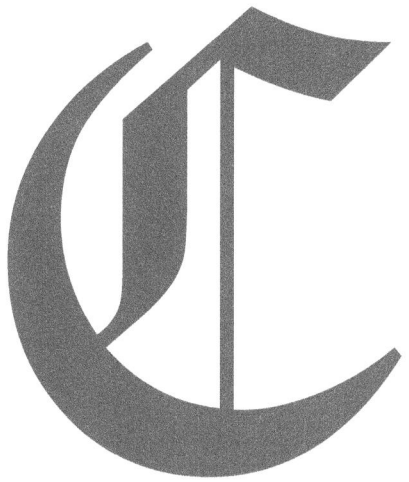

Carefulness

- Watch your tongue and keep your mouth shut, and you will stay out of trouble.

- It is not what you say that matters, but how you say it.

- I celebrate the happiness of others and find their joy and inspiration.

- I am here for a limited amount of time, and I am making the most of each and every moment granted to me.

Caution

- Caution is what we call cowardice in others.

- A railroad crossing is a place where it's better to be dead-sure than sure-dead.

- Be cautious in choosing friends, and be even more cautious in changing them.

- Caution is a good risk to take.

- A person can save himself from many hard falls by refraining from jumping to the conclusion.

- When we're afraid, we say we're cautious. When others are afraid, we say they're cowardly.

CHANGE

- Some people continue to change jobs, mates, and friends but never think of changing themselves.

- One cannot change yesterday, but can only make the most of today, and look with hope toward tomorrow; forget the past. Do well in the present and, in that way, prepare for the future.

- Change brings freshness.

- Change is the only constant in life.

- Social change is better achieved by being for something than against something.

- There is nothing that existed in your past that cannot be changed now. You are the creator of the past and the future. Therefore, you create the whole now, even the things that you feel are unchangeable. – *Kyron*

- You may realize that you see things not as they are but as you think they should be. Strive to change the things in yourself that you want to change in others. – *Keith D. Harrell*

- Constant change is here to stay.

- New ideas hurt some minds the same way new shoes hurt some feet.

- Most people are willing to change, not because they see the light, but because they feel the heat.

- The price of progress is change, and it is taking just about all we have.

- We can only change the world by changing men.

- We are the change we have been waiting for. – *Barack Obama*

- When you accept the fact that the only constant is change, you'll no longer be willing to do damage to yourself and others by refusing to accept it. Welcoming change is welcoming life. – *Anne Wilson Schaef*

Character

- Be big enough to admit and admire the abilities of people who are better than you are.

- Where we go and what we do advertises who we are.

- Character cannot be purchased, bargained for, inherited, rented, or imported from afar. It must be homegrown. – *Stephen Covey*

- It's not the load that breaks you down, it's the way you carry it. – *Lou Holtz*

- You can easily judge the character of a man by how he treats those who can do nothing for him. – *Malcolm S. Forbes*

- Character is made by many acts; it may be lost by a single one. – *Aristotle*

- Think right, act right, it is what you think and do that makes you what you are.

- It is not by a man's purse but by his character that he is rich or poor.

- Brains and beauty are nature's gifts; character is your own achievement.

- The measure of a man's character is not what he gets from his ancestors but what he leaves to his descendants.

- Take care of your character and your reputation will take care of itself.

- Men of genius are admired; men of wealth are envied; men of power are feared; but only men of character are trusted. – *Alfred Adler*

- A man may be better than his creed, his company, or his conduct. But no man is better than his character.

- You can no more blame your circumstances for your character than you can blame the mirror for the way you look.

- Ability will enable a man to get to the top, but it takes character to keep him there. – *American Proverb*

- People determine your character by observing what you stand for, fall for, and lie for.

- Youth and beauty fade; character endures forever.

- It isn't how high you go in life that counts, but how you get there.

- Some men succeed because of what they know, others because of what they do, and a few because of who they are.

- Character starts in cobwebs but ends in chains.

CHARITY

- Charity begins at home, and generally dies from a lack of outdoor exercise.

- Charity is twice blessed — it blesses the one who gives and the one who receives.

- Unless a man is a recipient of charity, he should be a contributor to it.

- Charity is the sterilized milk of human kind.

- True character means helping those you have every reason to believe would not help you.

- Sincere charity is the desire to be useful to others without any thought of recompense.

- If you don't have any charity in your heart, you have the worst kind of heart trouble. – *Bob Hope*

- It is more blessed to give than to receive. – *Acts 20: 35 KJV*

- The bee is more honored than others, not because she labors, but because she labors for others. – *St. John*

- The fragrance is always in the hand that gives the rose. – *Heda Bejar*

CHOICE

- I can be happy or unhappy. The choice is mine.

- Where in your life are you avoiding choices? Are you willing to make self-honoring choices today? If you don't make clear and concise choices, you'll be stuck with whatever shows up. – *Iyanla Vanzant*

- Choice, not chance, determines destiny.

- The choice is simple — you can either stand up and be counted, or lie down and be counted out.

- It is much wiser to choose what you say than to say what you choose.

- No one can grow by allowing others to make their decisions for them.

- Nothing great was ever done without an act of decision.

- Be cautious in choosing friends, and be even more cautious in changing them.

- If fate hands you lemons, try to make lemonade.

- Wise people sometimes change their minds, fools never.

- The universe totally supports every thought you choose to think and to believe. You have unlimited choices about what to think. Choose balance, harmony, and peace and express it in your life. – *Louise L. Hay*

CIRCUMSTANCES

- Bloom where you are planted. – *Mother Jones*

- Make yesterday's mistakes for your lessons.
- Don't rob the poor just because you can, or exploit the needy in court.
- What we see depends mainly on what we look for.

COMMITMENT

- Reconsider a commitment. You have the right to change your mind. – *Cheryl Richardson*
- What you dismiss as an ordinary coincidence may be an opening to an extraordinary adventure. – *Deepak Chopra, MD*
- Alone we do so little; together we can do so much.
- Noble deeds and hot baths are the best cures for depression. – *Dodie Smith*

Commonsense

- Commonsense is the knack of seeing things as they are and doing things as they ought to be done.

- An unusual amount of common sense is sometimes called wisdom.

- Emotion makes the world go round, but common sense keeps it from going too fast.

- Money. It's a good servant but a bad master. – *Gretchen Rubin, The Happiness Project*

Community

- Alone we do so little; together we can do so much.

- It takes a village to raise a child.

- I make an effort to connect and stay connected to loving friends and family because positive people add to my happiness.

Compassion

- Look at the weaknesses of others with compassion, not accusation. It's not what they're doing or should be doing that's the issue. The issue is your own shows in response to the situation and what you should be doing. – *Stephen R. Covey*

- Practice the healing power of a compassionate mind. Open your heart to other people without judgement, and radiate the message of delight at having them in your life. – *Caroline Myss and Peter Occhiogrosso*

- If passion drives you, let reason hold the reins.

- Treat everyone and everything with loving compassion. When you see no difference between the sacred and the profane, the saint or the sinner, that is the ultimate wisdom. – *Daniel Levin*

- Do not rejoice at my grief, for when mine is old, yours will be new. – *Spanish Proverb*

- The dew of compassion is a tear. – *George Gordon Byron*

Complaint

- Complaining is the thing to try when all else fails.

- One of the easiest things to find is fault.

- The person who is always finding fault seldom finds anything else.

- Before finding fault with another person, stop and count ten of your own.

- Faultfinding is as dangerous as it is easy.

- An expert faultfinder has no reason to be proud of his accomplishment.

- Don't find fault with what you don't think there was a reward for.

- When it comes to spotting the faults of others, everybody seems to have 20/20 vision.

- We do not get rid of our faults by calling attention to the faults of others.

Compliments

- A compliment a day keeps divorce far, far away.

- The highest compliment our patients can give us is the referral of their friends and family. Thank you for your truest. – *Eye Exam Clinic, Vicksburg, MS*

- A compliment is the soft soap that wipes out a dirty look.

- It is all right to always be looking for compliments to give to somebody else.

Compromise

- A compromise is the art of dividing a cake in such a way that everybody believes he got the biggest piece.

- A compromise is a deal in which two people get what neither of them wanted.

- Compromise is always wrong when it means sacrificing a principle.

- Peace won by the compromise of principles is a short-lived achievement.

Conceit

- A conceited person never gets anywhere because he thinks he is already there.

- A person who thinks too much of himself isn't thinking enough.

- Conceit is the only disease known to man that makes everybody sick except the person who has it.

- Conceit may puff a man up, but it never props him up.

- Give some people authority, and they will grow; give it to others, and they will swell.

- He who falls in love with himself will have no rivals.

- Heads that are filled with knowledge and wisdom have little space left for conceit.

- Nature abhors a vacuum. When a head lacks brains, nature fills it with conceit.

- One of the most difficult secrets for a man to keep is his opinion of himself.

- Pat others on the back, not yourself.

- Some men achieve greatness. Others are born great, and a few have greatness thrust upon them. The rest of us just think we're great.

- Talk to a man about himself, and he will listen for hours.

- The best remedy for conceit is to sit down and make a list of all the things you don't know.

- The fellow who gets on a high horse is riding for a fall.

- The greatest fault is to be conscious of none.

- The man who believes in nothing but himself lives in a very small world.

- The person who knows everything has a lot to learn.

- The strength that comes from confidence can be quickly lost in conceit.

- There's more hope for a confessed sinner than for a conceited saint.

- Being unusually pleased with yourself is the surest way of offending everybody else.

Condemnation

- Speak not against anyone whose burden you have not weighed yourself. – *Marion Bradley*

- One man cannot hold another man down in the ditch without remaining down in the ditch with him. – *Booker T. Washington*

- If you judge people you have no time to love them. – *Mother Teresa*

Confidence

- You must first be a believer if you want to be an achiever.

- Confidence is the feeling you have before you fully understand the situation.

- Faith gives us the courage to face the present with confidence and the future with expectancy.

- A good leader inspires men to have confidence in him; a great leader inspires them to have confidence in themselves.

- A wise man is never confused by what he can't understand, but a fool is sure to be.

- An expert can take something you already know and make it sound confusing.

- An expert is always able to create confusion out of simplicity.

- Many people look ahead; some look back, but most look confused.

- Belief in yourself is more important than endless worries of what others think of you. – *Ngugi Wa Thiong'o*

- A man who wants to lead the orchestra must turn his back on the crowd. – *Anonymous*

- Shoot for the moon. Even if you miss it, you will land among the stars. – *Les Brown*

- If you don't have confidence, you'll always find a way not to win. – *Carl Lewis*

- God is the one that you remember and get confidence in.

- It is a funny thing about life; if you refuse to accept anything but the best, you very often get it.

- If you're doing the right thing, if you're not harming yourself or others, you need not be concerned with what others think. You're free! – *Brian L Weiss, MD*

- Only when you are no longer afraid do we begin to live.

- We have to dare to be ourselves, however frightening or strange that self may prove to be.

- If you've made up your mind that you can do something, you're absolutely right.

- He like a rock in the sea, unshaken, stands his ground. – *Mother Teresa*

Confrontation

- The next time you have a disagreement or confrontation with someone, attempt to understand that person's concerns. Address these issues in a creative and mutually beneficial way. – *Stephen R. Covey*

- He who speaks of others' failures with happiness, will hear of his own with bitterness.

- Those who mock the poor insult their Maker; those who rejoice at the misfortune of others will be punished. – *Proverbs 17:5*

Conscience

- A clear conscience fears no accusation. – *African Proverb*

- A man's best boss is a well-trained conscience.

- A man's conscience tells him what he shouldn't do — but it does not keep him from doing it. – *Frank A. Clark*

- A man's conscience, and not his mattress, has most to do with his sleep.

- Conscience is like a baby. It has to go to sleep before you can. – *Harvey Mackay*

- Conscience is the only mirror that doesn't flatter.

- Conscience keeps more people awake than coffee. – *Arnold Glasow*

- Happiness is a healthy mental attitude, a grateful spirit, a clear conscience, and a heart full of love.

- Happy is the man who renounces everything that places a strain on his conscience.

- It is a sermon that pricks the conscience. It must have good points.

- It is your conscience that warns you to be careful about what it can't stop you from doing.

- One should be more concerned about what his conscience whispers than about what other people shout.

- The best tranquilizer is a good conscience. – *Benjamin Franklin*

- The greatest tormentor of the human soul is a guilty conscience.

- The testimony of a good conscience is worth more than that of a character witness.

- Those who remember the past with a clear conscience need have no fear of the future.

- Thousands of people become hard of hearing when conscience speaks.

- To know what is right and not to do it is as bad as doing it wrong.

- Your conscience doesn't really keep you from doing anything; it merely keeps you from enjoying it.

Consistency

- Are you willing to stop "people-pleasing" today? The best way to honor yourself is to say no.

- When you say no, and yes only when you really want to say yes! – *Iyanla Vanzant*

- Anything worth doing is worth doing well.

- Be as constant as the north star.

Contentment

- Contentment in life consists not of great wealth but of simple wants.

- Contentment is a matter of hoping for the best and making the best of what we get.

- Contentment is often the result of being too lazy to stir up a fuss.

- Contentment is something that depends a little on position and a lot on disposition.

- Contentment is when your earning power equals your yearning power.

- Happiness is in the heart, not in the circumstances.

- If you can't be content with what you have received, be thankful for what you have escaped. – *Izaak Walton*

- It is right to be contented with what we have, never with what we are. – *James Mackin*

- Patience, forbearance, and understanding are companions to contentment.

- The best way for a person to have a contented state of mind is for him to count his blessings, not his cash.

- The godly eat to their hearts' content, but the bellies of the wicked go hungry. – *Proverbs 13:25*

CONTROL

- Trying to limit anybody about anything defies the laws of the Universe. It cannot be done. You cannot control others, but you can control and create your own reality. – *Abraham Hicks*

- You are the only person who has control over your eating habits. You can always resist something if you choose to. – *Louise L. Hay*

- You can only control your reactions and attitudes to what happens to you. You cannot control the actual events. Learn the difference. – *Brian L. Weiss, M.D.*

- I cannot change the past and I cannot predict the future, but I can control the moment and enjoy it before it becomes the past.

- I control myself from buying things that are beyond my means.

- Sensible people control their temper, they earn respect by overlooking wrongs. – *Proverbs 19:11*

- Those who control their tongue will have a long life; opening your mouth can ruin everything.

Contrition

- Jesus Lord, I ask for mercy. Let me not implore in vain. All my sins are now detested. Never will I sin again. – *God of Mercy and Compassion (I)*

- If your relationship with God is injured, apologize today for your attitudes and thoughts. Tell God you have misunderstood His actions and badly misjudged His character. Tell Him exactly how you felt and why, and ask Him for His forgiveness. – *Dr. Bruce Wilkinson*

- When a friend makes a mistake, don't rub it in. Rub it out.

Conversation

- An intelligent conversationalist is one who nods his head in agreement while you're talking.

- Conversation is an exercise of the mind, but gossiping is merely an exercise of the tongue.

- Fascinating conversation is the art of telling people a little less than they want to know.

- If you are not a charming conversationalist, you may still be a big hit as a charmed listener.

- If you wish to get along with people, pretend not to know already whatever they are telling. – *Vikrant*

- The real art of conversation is not only saying the right thing in the right place, but to leave unsaid the wrong thing at the tempting moment. – *Dorothy Nevill*

- ❦ The true spirit of conversation consists in building on another man's observation, not overturning it. – *Edward G Bulwer-Lytton*

- ❦ The secret of polite conversation is never to open your mouth unless you have something to say.

Conviction

- ❦ Conviction is a belief that you hold or that holds you.

- ❦ Say yes until you believe it.

- ❦ Right is right, even if everyone is against it, and wrong is wrong, even if everyone is for it. – *William Penn*

- ❦ Ah, but a man's reach should exceed his grasp, or what's a heaven for? – *Robert Browning*

- ❦ Winning isn't everything, but it beats anything that comes in second. – *Paul "Bear" Bryant*

- ❦ People generally have too many opinions and not enough convictions.

- ❦ If you don't stand for something, you will likely fall for anything.

- Be bold in what you stand for, but careful in what you fall for.

- The true measure of a man is the height of his ideals, the breadth of his sympathy, the depth of his convictions, and the length of his patience.

- Whether you think you can, or you think you can't, you are right. – *Henry Ford*

COOPERATION

- Cooperation is doing what I tell you to do and doing it quickly.

- Everybody likes friendly attention and cooperation. We always get it when we give it.

- If you don't think cooperation is necessary, watch what happens to a wagon if one wheel comes off.

- No one can whistle a symphony. It takes an orchestra to play it. – *H.E. Luccock*

Correction

- Mockers hate to be corrected, so they stay away from the wise. – *Proverbs 15:12*

- Anyone who rebukes a mocker will get an insult in return. Anyone who corrects the wicked will get hurt. – *Proverbs 9:7*

- So don't bother correcting mockers; they will only hate you. But correct the wise, and they will love you. – *Proverbs 9:8*

Counseling

- Plans fail for lack of counsel, but with many advisers they succeed. – *Proverbs 15:22*

- In giving advice, I advise you, be short. – *Horace*

- He who builds to every man's advice will have a crooked house. – *Danish Proverb*

- It is easy to give good advice to the sick. – *Terence*

- To attempt to advise conceited people is like whistling against the wind. – *Thomas Hood*

- Talk low, talk slow and don't say too much. – *John Wayne*

COURAGE

- The truest test of moral courage is the ability to ignore an insult.

- The courage to speak must be matched by the wisdom to listen. – *Charles McKenzie*

- Be bold in what you stand for but careful in what you fall for.

- Remember, you are your own doctor when it comes to curing cold feet.

- Courage is not the absence of fear, but the conquest of it. – *Brett McKay*

- Many a man who is proud of his right to say what he pleases wishes he had the courage to do so.

- Courage is the quality it takes to look at yourself with candor, your adversaries with kindness, and your setbacks with serenity.

- Keep your fears to yourself, but share your courage with others. – *Robert Louis Stevenson*

- Freedom is the sure possession of only those who have the courage to defend it. – *Pericles*

- Prayer gives strength to the weak, faith to the fainthearted, and courage to the fearful.

- The test of courage comes when you are in the minority; the test of tolerance comes when you are in the majority. – *Ralph W. Sockman*

- The only thing we have to fear is fear itself. – *Franklin D. Roosevelt*

- Pain nourishes courage. You can't be brave if you've only had wonderful things happen to you. – *Mary Tyler Moore*

- Often the test of courage is not to die, but to live. – *Vittorio Alfieri*

- Cowards die many times before their death; the valiant never taste of death but once. – *William Shakespeare*

- Once bitten, twice shy. – *Julian Barnes*

- Find the courage to ask for what you want. Others have the right to tell you yes or no, but you always have the right to ask. Likewise, everybody has the right to ask you for what they want, and you have the right to say yes or no. – *Don Miguel Ruiz*

- Help others quietly, without expecting gratitude or rewards. Let the healing power of your spirit run through your hand as you reach to touch another, but say nothing to the person you help. I learned that courage was not the absence of fear but the triumph over it. The brave man is not he who does not feel afraid, but he who conquers that fear.

- Courage If you're evolving into a more loving, more compassionate, less violent person, then you're moving in the right direction. – *Brian L. Weiss, M.D.*

- Life shrinks or expands in proportion to one's courage. – *Anais Nin*

CRIME

- A crooked path is the shortest way to the penitentiary.

- A juvenile delinquent usually prefers vice to advice.

- A shady business never produces a sunny life. – *B.C. Forbes*

- Crime begins in the mind. A man has to think wrong before he acts wrong.

- Gossip is one form of crime for which the law provides no punishment.

- The best way to put down crime is to stop putting up with it.

- The death penalty may not eliminate crime, but it stops repeaters.

CRITICISM

- A person usually criticizes the individual whom he secretly envies.

- A valuable friend is one who'll tell you what you should be told, even if it momentarily offends you.

- Adverse criticism from a wise man is more to be desired than the enthusiastic approval of a fool. – *American salesman*

- Any fool can criticize, condemn, and complain — and most fools do. – *Dale Carnegie*

- Criticism from a friend is better than flattery from an enemy.

- Criticism is like dynamite. It has its place, but should be handled only by experts.

- Criticism is the disapproval of people, not for having faults, but for having faults different from your own.

- Don't criticize the other fellow's plan unless you have a better one to offer.

- Envy is blind and knows nothing except to depreciate the excellence of others.

- If you are afraid of criticism, you'll die doing nothing.

- It is usually best to be generous with praise, but cautious with criticism.

- Never fear criticism when you're right; never ignore criticism when you're wrong.

- No one appreciates the value of constructive criticism more thoroughly than the one who's giving it. – *Hal Chadwick*

- One of the hardest things to take is one of the easiest things to give—criticism.

- One of the surest marks of good character is a man's ability to accept personal criticism without feeling malice toward the one who gives it. – *O.A. Battista*

- The best way to lose a friend is to tell him something for his own good.

- You might possibly avoid criticism by saying nothing, doing nothing, and being nothing.

- Whoever stubbornly refuses to accept criticism will suddenly be destroyed beyond recovery. – *Proverbs 29:1*

- If you ignore criticism, you will end in poverty and disgrace; if you accept correction, you will be honored. – *Proverbs 13:18*

- If you listen to constructive criticism, you will be at home among the wise. – *Proverbs 15:31-32*

CURIOSITY

- Curiosity is nothing more than freewheeling intelligence.

- Enough curiosity may enable you to learn, but too much of it can get you into trouble.

- Nothing so excites a man's curiosity as a woman's complete silence.

- The things most people want to know about are usually none of their business. – *George Bernard Shaw*

- Be curious, not judgmental. – *Walt Whitman*

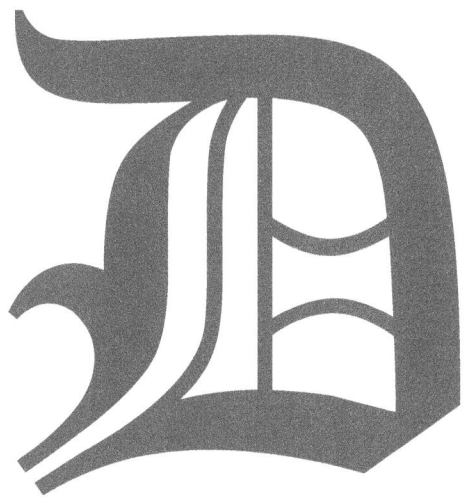

DEATH

- On his examination paper, a boy wrote, *"A natural death is where you die by yourself without a doctor's help."*

- There is a way that seems right to a man, but in the end it leads to death. – *Proverb 14:12*

- A person can survive almost everything except death.

- Be as kind as you can today; tomorrow you may not be here.

- Death is the beginning of the end. – *A Rainbow of Hope*

- Death is the golden key that opens the palace of eternity. – *John Milton*

- Make this your motto: Don't die until you are dead. – *Billy Connolly*

- Other appointments in life we can neglect or break, but death is an appointment that no man can ignore, no man can break. – *Billy Graham*

- ❦ The nearer the time comes for our departure from this life, the greater our regret for wasting so much of it.

- ❦ The one thing certain about life is that we must leave it.

- ❦ The only thing worse than growing old is to be denied the privilege.

- ❦ We go to the grave of a friend, saying, *"A man is dead,"* but angels throng about him, saying, *"A man is born."* – *Henry Ward Beecher*

- ❦ When we die, we leave behind us all that we have and take with us all that we are.

- ❦ Don't face death without facing God. Don't even speak of death without speaking to God. He and He alone can guide you through the valley. And only God is committed to getting you there safely. – *Max Lucado*

DEBTS

- ❦ A good salesman can talk you into debt.

- America may be the land of the free, but not the debt-free.

- Creditors have better memories than debtors. – *Benjamin Franklin*

- Debt is like quicksand, and it is just about as hard to get out of.

- Debts of gratitude are the most difficult to collect.

- Many who are quick to run into debt find it takes a long time to crawl out.

- Some friends stick together until debt does them part.

- The doorway out of debt opens a little bit further with each payment you make toward yesterday, which is also a payment toward tomorrow. – *Suze Orman*

- The man who borrows trouble is always in debt.

- What you don't own won't hurt you.

- Yesterday's luxuries are today's debts.

- Being debt-free makes me happy.

DEEDS

- Kind words can never die, but without kind deeds they can sound mighty sick.

- You always remember a kind deed, particularly if it was yours.

- Small deeds done are better than great deeds planned. – *Peter Marshall*

- Do good deeds ever get dizzy from doing too many good turns?

- It is vain to use words when deeds are expected.

DEFEAT

- Many things are worse than defeat, and compromise with evil is one of them.

- Defeat is simply a signal to press onward. – *Helen Keller*

- ❦ Defeat never comes to any man until he admits it. – *Josephus Daniels*

- ❦ The highway of fear is the shortest route to defeat.

DESTINY

- ❦ Destiny is no matter of chance. It is a matter of choice. – *William Jennings Bryan*

- ❦ Our destiny is largely in our hands. – *Frederick Douglass*

- ❦ What chance can a man have to control his destiny when he can't control himself?

DETERMINATION

- ❦ The difference between a successful person and others is not a lack of strength, not a lack of knowledge, but rather a lack of will. – *Vince Lombardi*

- ❦ I will work until my good becomes better and my better becomes my best.

- It is never too late to be what you might have been. – *George Elliot*

- Nothing is difficult for those who have the will.

- The difference between the impossible and the possible lies in a person's determination. – *Tommy Lasorda*

- The truest wisdom is a resolute determination. – *Napoleon Bonaparte*

- If you've made up your mind you can do something, you're absolutely right. –*Woodrow Wilson*

- Stand for something or you will fall for anything. – *Rosa Parks*

Dexterity

- You must not only aim right, but draw the bow with all your might. – *Henry David Thoreau*

- The difference between ordinary and extraordinary is that little "extra." Today, demand more of yourself than you or anyone else can expect. – *Keith D. Harrell*

- Success today requires the agility and drive to rethink, react, and reinvent. – *Bill Gates*

DIFFICULTIES

- A cool head may sometimes keep a man out of trouble, but more often, it's cold feet.

- A lot of trouble arises from workers who don't think and from thinkers who don't work.

- Despite all the pain and trouble, life is still better than any alternative.

- Don't make your friends a dumping ground for your troubles.

- If you would like to know who is responsible for more of your troubles, take a look in the mirror.

- In the middle of difficulty lies opportunity. – *Albert Einstein*

- Invite trouble, and it will usually come.

- It is not so much the greatness of our troubles, as the littleness of our spirit, which makes us complain. – *James Hudson Taylor*

- Most of our troubles arise from loafing when we should be working and talking when we should be listening.

- Most of us listen to the troubles of other people just for the chance to get back at them with our own.

- Patience is the greatest of all shock absorbers. About the only thing you can get in a hurry is trouble. – *Lord Thomas R. Dewar*

- Tackle any difficulty at first sight, for the longer you gaze at it, the bigger it grows.

- The difficulties of life are intended to make us better, not bitter.

- The man who smiles in the face of trouble is either brave or covered by insurance.

- There are a lot of people who get into trouble trying to keep up with the Joneses, especially the Dow Joneses.

- Troubles and weeds thrive on lack of attention. - Attentiveness vs. Distraction" – *Presentation, Domenic Hoople*

- Worry is interest paid on trouble before it becomes due. – *William R. Inge*

DIGNITY

- It has been said that dignity is the ability to hold back from the tongue that which never should have been on the mind in the first place.

- Dignity is a mask we wear to hide our ignorance. – *Elbert Hubbard*

- Dignity is one thing that cannot be preserved in alcohol. – *American Proverb*

DIPLOMACY

- Diplomacy is convincing a man he's a liar without actually saying so.

- ⚜ Diplomacy is the art of making others believe that you believe what you don't believe.

- ⚜ Diplomacy is the art of saying things in such a way that nobody knows exactly what you mean.

- ⚜ Diplomacy is the art of taking sides without anyone knowing it.

- ⚜ Diplomacy is to do and say the nastiest things in the nicest way. – *Isaac Goldberg*

DIRECTION

- ⚜ The great thing in this world is not so much where we are, but in what direction we are moving. – *Oliver Wendell Holmes Sr.*

- ⚜ I enjoy my life's journey, wherever it takes me, for that is the only trip that I can fully embrace.

- ⚜ I know the direction in which I am marching, although I am not the master of the means.

- Do not go where the path may lead, go instead where there is no path and leave a trail. – *Ralph Waldo Emerson*

DISAGREEMENT

- It's better to disagree than agree and all be wrong.

- The only way to settle a disagreement is on the basis of what's right, not who's right.

- It's annoying when people disagree with you, especially when you're right.

DISCIPLINE

- A really good parent is a provider, a counselor, an adviser, and, when necessary, a disciplinarian.

- Character does not reach its best until it is controlled, harnessed, and disciplined.

- Discipline yourself and others won't need to. – *John Wooden*

- If you reject discipline, you only harm yourself, but if you listen to correction, you grow in understanding. – *Proverbs 15:32*

- My child, don't reject the Lord's discipline, and don't be upset when he corrects you. – *Proverbs 3:11 NLT*

- Never strike a child! You might miss and hurt yourself.

- People who accept discipline are on the pathway to life, but those who ignore correction will go astray. – *Proverbs 10:17 NLT*

- Take yourself and your creative life seriously. Make time for self-expression. Be disciplined. This is the way to develop your unique gifts and talents. – *Christiane Northrup, M.D.*

- Those who spare the rod of discipline hate their children. Those who love their children care enough to discipline them. – *Proverbs 13:24*

- To learn, you must love discipline; it is stupid to hate correction. – *Proverbs 12:1 NLT*

- What kids need today is plenty of LSD — Love, Security, and Discipline.

- Willpower cannot be furnished by anyone but you.

DOUBT

- If you doubt the propriety of doing a thing, you'd better give yourself the benefit of the doubt and not do it.

- Many people believe their doubts, and doubt their beliefs.

- No one can live in doubt when he has prayed in faith.

- When in doubt, don't. – *Benjamin Franklin*

- When in doubt, tell the truth. – *Mark Twain*

DREAMS

- Inbetween yesterday's regret and tomorrow's dream is today's opportunity. Seize the chance! – *Ifeanyi Enoch Onuoha*

- Don't be unhappy if your dreams never come true; just be thankful your nightmares don't.

- It is pleasant to see dreams come true, but fools refuse to turn from evil to attain them. – *Proverbs 13:19, NLT*

- Those who think they are dreamers are usually just sleepers.

- A man's dreams are an index to his greatness. – *Zadok Rabinwitz*

DUTY

- You can do anything you ought to do.

- Duty is a task we look forward to with distaste, perform with reluctance, and brag about afterwards. – *HJW III*

- We stood where duty required us to stand. – *Breoh Jr.*

- Some folks who do their duty as they see it need to consult an eye specialist.

- An excuse is a statement given to cover up for a duty not well done or not done at all.

- Duty makes us do things well, but love makes us do them beautifully. – *Phillips Brooks*

- Happiness will never come your way as long as your back is turned on duty.

- Hard work and devotion to duty will surely get you a promotion, unless, of course, the boss has a relative who wants the job.

- To be humble to superiors is a duty, to equals courtesy, to inferiors nobleness. – *Benjamin Franklin*

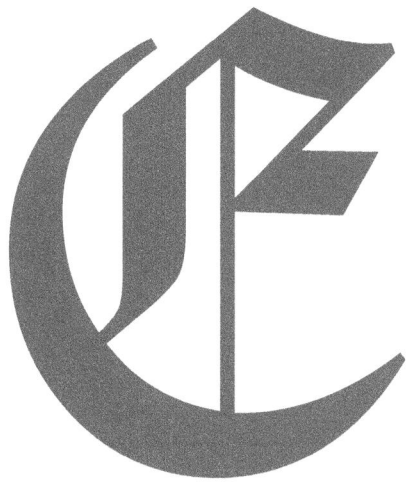

Economy

- Many people don't start economizing until they run out of money.

- Don't cheat the Lord and call it "economy."

- Economizing is easier when you're broke.

- If you want economy, never let an economic question get into politics.

- Most people might practice economy if they had something left to practice with.

- The only thing wrong with our economy is that nobody wants to economize.

- The trouble with today's managed economy is the mismanagement.

- The way the American economy is going, we'll soon have a system of checks and bounces.

- There comes a time when a nation, as well as an individual, must choose between tightening the belt or losing the pants.

Education

- A little learning may be a dangerous thing, but it's still safer than total ignorance.

- Education is an ornament in prosperity and a refuge in adversity. – *Aristotle*

- Education is knowing what you want, knowing where to get it, and knowing what to do with it after you get it.

- Education is not a head full of facts, but knowing how and where to find them.

- Education is not received. It is achieved. – *Albert Einstein*

- Education is one commodity for which we can never have a surplus.

- Education means developing the mind, not stuffing the memory.

- Education should include knowledge of what to do with it.

- It is a thousand times better to have common sense without education than to have education without common sense. – *Robert Green Ingersoll*

- It's not what is poured into a student that counts, but what is planted. – *Linda Conway*

- It's what you learn after you know it all that counts. – *John Wooden*

- No man is fully educated until he learns to read himself.

- Not all educated people are intelligent.

- The least expensive education is to profit from the mistakes of others and ourselves.

- The only known cure for ignorance is education.

- The roots of education are bitter, but the fruit is sweet. – *Aristotle*

- The true object of education should be to train one to think clearly and act rightly.

- The truly educated man is that rare individual who can distinguish between reality and illusion.

- You can buy education, but wisdom is a gift that can never be. – *Oscar Auliq Ice*

- Your graduation is just the beginning of a wonderful future for bright and talented people like you; you'll surely reach your goals and achieve much success ahead.

EGO

- An egotist is a person who is his own best friend. – *Evan Esar*

- An egotist is an inferior person with a superiority complex.

- Egotism is a disease that often kills men before they know they have it.

- Egotism is obesity of the head.

- Egotism is partly enthusiasm but mostly ignorance.

- Egotism is the glue with which you get stuck in yourself. – *Dan Post*

- No matter what effect the egotist has on others, he always fascinates himself.

- The most difficult secret for a man to keep is his own opinion of himself. – *Marcel Pagnol*

- Pride hides a man's faults to himself and magnifies them to everyone else. – *Chronicles 12:7*

- Some of us veer to the left, and some of us swing to the right, but most of us are self-centered.

- Some people are so egotistical that every time they look in the mirror, they take a bow.

- The emptiest man is in sore need of surgery; they need about half of their ego removed.

- The eyes of an egotist look in instead of out.

- The more praise a man is willing to take, the less he deserves it.

- The more you speak of yourself, the more you are likely to lie. – *Johann Georg Zimmermann*

- The more you talk about yourself, the more apt you are to lie.

- The only time some people don't interrupt is when you're praising them.

- The strange thing is that man is satisfied with so little in himself but demands so much from others.

- When a man tries himself, the verdict is usually in his favor.

- When you lay your ego aside and return to that from which you originally emanated, you'll begin to immediately see the power of intention working with, for, and through you in a multitude of ways. – *Dr. Wayne W. Dyer*

ENCOURAGEMENT

- A friend will strengthen you with his prayers, bless you with his love, and encourage you with his hope.

- Keep your ideals high enough to inspire you and low enough to encourage you.

- Pat others on the back, not yourself.

- The best thing to do behind a person's back is pat it.

Endurance

- The weak fall, but the strong will remain and never go under! – *Anne Frank*

- Sorrow is a fruit. God does not make it grow on limbs too weak to bear it. – *Victor Hugo*

- Strength does not come from physical capacity. It comes from an indomitable will. – *Mahatma Gandhi*

Enemies

- A man's reputation is a blend of what his friends, enemies, and acquaintances say behind his back.

- A still tongue makes no enemies.

- Anyone who's written an autobiography learns you can make two kinds of enemies with such a book — the people you mention and those you don't.

- As long as your conscience is your friend, never mind about your enemies.

- It sometimes looks foolish for folks to be spending so much time loving their enemies when they should be treating their friends a little better.

- Kindness is the ability to treat your enemy decently.

- Love your enemies, but if you really want to make them mad, ignore them completely.

- Mankind's worst enemy is fear of work! – *Napoleon Bonaparte*

- No enemy is more dangerous than a friend who isn't quite sure whether he's for you or against you.

- Nobody can have too many friends, but one enemy may constitute a surplus.

- People make enemies by complaining too much to their friends.

- The difference between our friends and our enemies is this: Our friends love us in spite of our faults, and our enemies hate us in spite of our virtues.

- There is only one reason why your enemy can't become your friend — YOU!

- We make more enemies by what we say than friends by what we do. – *John Collins*

- When you bury the hatchet, don't bury it in your enemy's back.

- You can meet friends everywhere, but you can't meet enemies anywhere — you have to make them.

Enjoyment

- Don't expect to enjoy life if you keep your milk of human kindness all bottled up.

- Enjoy today and don't waste it grieving over a bad yesterday — tomorrow may be even worse.

- Enjoy yourself. These are the "good old days" you're going to miss in the years ahead.

- If you don't enjoy what you have, how could you be happier with more?

- Not what we have, but what we enjoy, constitutes our abundance. – *Epicurus*

- The good things of life were made to enjoy. Enjoying a thing means sharing it with others.

- Your conscience doesn't really keep you from doing anything, it mere keeps you from enjoying it.

ENTHUSIASM

- You cannot run faster than your legs can carry you.

- A healthy mind in a healthy body; a healthy voice in a healthy body. – *Henry David Thoreau*

- Enthusiasm for hard work is more sincerely expressed by the person who is paying for it.

- Enthusiasm is a good engine, but it needs intelligence for a driver. – *Woody Allen*

- Enthusiasm is contagious — and so is the lack of it. – *Suzanne Wood Fisher, Amish Proverbs*

- He who has no fire in himself cannot warm others.

- None are so old as those who have cultivated enthusiasm. – *Henry David Thoreau*

- The gap between enthusiasm and indifference is filled with failures. – *Mencius*

- Years wrinkle the skin, but lack of enthusiasm wrinkles the soul.

- Enthusiasm without knowledge is no good; haste makes mistake. – *Proverbs 19:2*

ENVY

- Don't mind the fellow who belittles you; he's only trying to cut you down to his size. – *Dexter Yager*

- Envy is usually the mother of gossip.

- Envy provides the mud that failure throws at success.

- Love is the glue that cements friendship; jealousy keeps it from sticking.

- Love looks through a telescope; envy, through a microscope. – *Josh Billings*

- One blessing in being poor, honest, and hardworking is that nobody envies you.

- Sometimes criticism is nothing but a mild form of envy.

- The sunlight of love will kill all the germs of jealousy and hate.

- There are many roads to hate, but envy is one of the shortest of them all.

- We underrate that which we do not possess.

EQUALITY

- A sure cure for conceit is visiting a cemetery, and discovering that eggheads and boneheads get equal billing. – *Bernie Hughes*

- There's justice for all, but it doesn't seem to be equally distributed.

- Give everyone equal status in your mind because it will prepare you to learn from everyone.

- Equal opportunity means everyone will have a fair chance at being incompetent. – *Laurence J. Peter*

EVIL

- Evil wins when the good don't fight.

- Evil people are eager for rebellion, but they will be severely punished. – *Proverbs 17:11*

- If you repay good with evil, evil will never leave your house. – *Proverbs 17:13*

- Don't envy evil people or desire their company. – *Proverbs 24:1*

- The only thing necessary for the triumph of evil is for good men to do nothing. – *Edmund Burke*

- When you choose the lesser of two evils, always remember that it is still an evil. –*Max Lerner*

- Pity the criminal all you like, but don't call evil good. – *Feodor Dostoevski*

- Evil often triumphs but it never conquers. – *J. Roux*

- Hear no evil, see no evil, speak no evil. – *Legend related to the "Three Wise Monkeys"*

Excellence

- The quality of a person's life is in direct proportion to his commitment to excellence, regardless of his chosen field of endeavor.

- Excellence is not an accomplishment. It is a spirit, a never ending process. – *Lawrence Miller*

- We are what we repeatedly do. Excellence, then, is not an act but a habit. – *Aristotle*

Excesses

- There are definitely things you should not do to excess. For example, addictions that harm your physical body stop your soul's growth and cloud your direct rapport with God. Ask God to help strengthen your will and help you learn restraint. – *Sylvia Browne*

- Are your closets, drawers, and cabinets filled up with things that you never use? Get rid of the excess to make room for what you love. – *Julie Morgenstern*

- Clutter equals a state of being many; One man's clutter, is another man's treasure. – *St. Mary's Catholic Church Bulletin*

- Eliminate clutter from your home and work life to balance the flow of activities. – *Doreen Virtue, Ph.D.*

EXCUSES

- A flimsy excuse is one that your wife can see through.

- The real man is one who always finds excuses for others, but never excuses himself. – *Henry Ward Beecher*

- An excuse is a statement given to cover up for a duty not well done, or not done at all.

- Excuses fool no one but the person who makes them.

- Most failures are expert at making excuses.

- Never give an excuse that you would not be willing to accept.

- The man who really wants to do something finds a way; the other man finds an excuse.

- The most unprofitable item ever manufactured is an excuse. – *John Mason*

- Those who are most successful in making excuses have no energy left for anything else.

- When you don't want to do anything; one excuse is as good as another. – *Yiddish Proverb*

- Where in your life are you offering excuses for not standing in your power? Are you ready to eliminate excuses today? Excuses are means by which you avoid, deny and resist the greatness you know yourself to be. – *Iyanla Vanzant*

Exercise

- Digging for a fact is better mental exercise than jumping to a conclusion.

- If you don't move your body, your brain thinks you're dead. Movement of the body will not only clear out the "sludge," but will also give you more energy. Treat your body like a car—keep it tuned up and it will run for a very long time. – *Sylvia Browne*

- If you must exercise, why not exercise kindness?

- Jumping to conclusion is about the only exercise some people get.

- The best exercise is to exercise discretion at the dining table.

- Violent exercise after sixty is apt to be harmful — especially if you do it with a knife and fork.

- Whether or not the scientific research supports exercising as a way to achieve happiness. I am exercising today because it feels good and because research does confirm that exercise is good for my physical health.

- I feel happier exercising especially if the activity is something I love to do, like dancing or walking.

- I do happiness exercises to strengthen my joyful emotions just as I try to do physical exercises to improve my body.

- Walking a mile for a cigarette may be healthier than smoking one.

- Nurture your physical self by eating the right foods, getting sufficient rest and relaxation, and exercising on a regular basis. A good exercise program will build your body in three areas endurance, flexibility, and strength. – *Stephen R. Covey*

Expectations

- The best way to avoid disappointment is not to expect anything from anyone.

- Keep your expectations high on achievement and low on people.

- Don't expect too much. It is always better to feel surprised than to feel disappointed.

- If wishes were horses, beggars would ride. – *A Collection of Scottish Proverbs (1628)*

Experience

- A wise man learns by the experience of others. An ordinary man learns by his own experience. A fool learns by nobody's experience. – *American Proverb*

- You are the product of your experiences.

- Character grows in the soil of experience, with the fertilization of example, the moisture of desire, and the sunshine of satisfaction. – *Stephen Covey*

- Experience increases our wisdom but doesn't seem to reduce our follies. – *Josh Billings*

- Experience is a form of knowledge acquired in only two ways — by doing and by being done.

- Experience is the best teacher, and considering what it costs, it should be.

- Experience is what makes your mistakes so familiar.

- Experience is what prevents you from making the same mistake against in exactly the same way.

- Experience is what teaches you that you need a lot more.

- Experience is what tells you to watch your step, and it is also what you get if you don't.

- Experience makes a person better or bitter.

- If experience is the best teacher, many of us are mighty poor pupils.

- It requires experience to know how to use it.

- Our wisdom usually comes from our experience, and our experience comes largely from our foolishness. – *Sacha Guitry*

- Sixty-five is the age when one acquires sufficient experience to lose his job.

- Some people profit by their experiences, others never recover from them.

- The best advice you'll get is from someone who made the same mistake himself.

- There is no way to get experience except through experience.

- Trying to give people the benefit of your experience is one way of getting a lot more.

- You are the product of your experiences.

EXPERTS

- An expert is someone who doesn't know any more than you do but is better organized.

- The expert in anything was once a beginner. – *Helen Hayes*

- Never become so much of an expert that you stop gaining expertise. View life as a continuous learning experience. – *Denis Waitley*

Extravagance

- The remarkable thing about most of us is our ability to live beyond our means.

- The average man's ambition is to be able to afford what he's spending.

- Increased earnings nearly always lead to increased yearnings.

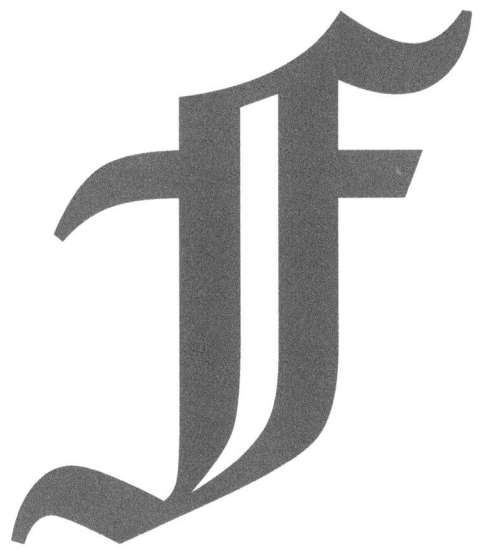

FACTS

- A failure is a man who has blundered, but is not able to cash in on the experience. – *Elbert Hubbard*

- A sure way to stop a red-hot argument is to lay a few cold facts on it.

- A thousand possibilities do not make one fact.

- Boasting and sleeping are the forerunners of failure.

- Digging for a fact is better mental exercise than jumping to a conclusion.

- Education is not a head full of facts, but knowing how and where to find facts.

- Every man has a right to his opinion, but no man has a right to be wrong about the facts. – *Bernard M. Baruch*

- Fact is fact and feeling is feeling; never does the second change the first.

- Facts are stubborn, but statistics are more pliable. – *Mark Twain*

- Facts are troublesome things to the evildoer.

- Facts do not cease to exist just because they are ignored. – *Aldous Huxley*

- Facts do not change; feelings do.

- Facts mean nothing unless they are rightly understood, rightly related, and rightly interpreted. – *William Jennings Bryan*

- Facts that are not frankly faced have a habit of stabbing us in the back. – *Harold Bowden*

FAILURE

- If you fail to plan, you are planning to fail. – *Benjamin Franklin*

- Failure is not the worst thing in the world. The very worst is not to try.

- Failure is only the opportunity to begin again more intelligently. – *Henry Ford*

- Failure is success if we can learn from it. – *Malcolm Probes*

- Failure always overtakes those who have the power to do without the will to act.

- Failure is not necessarily missing the target, but aiming too low.

- Failure is the path of least persistence.

- Failures are divided into those who thought and never did, and those who did and never thought. – *John Charles Salak*

- Fear of failure is the father of failure.

- Getting the facts is only half the job; the other half is to use them intelligently.

- It is easier to believe a lie that one has heard a thousand times than a fact no one ever heard before. – *Robert Lynd*

- It's easier to get facts than to face them.

- Many of life's failures are men who did not realize how close they were to success when they gave up. – *Thomas Edison*

- People should keep their mouths shut and their pens dry until they know the facts.

- The hardest thing about facts is to face them.

- The most prolific inventors are those who invent excuses for their failures.

- The only thing in life achieved without effort is failure. – *Francis of Assisi*

- The road to failure is greased with the slime of indifference.

- The train of failure usually runs on the track of laziness. – *Laziness leads to failure, The New Indian Express, Published: 27 th August 2010 | Last Updated: 16 th May*

- Wisdom is learned more from failure than from success. – *Samuel Smiles*

Faith

- Doubt makes the mountain which faith can move.

- When you cease to use your faith, you lose it.

- Have faith during inevitable conflict. Be willing to hang in there. You never know how something will turn out. – *Christiane Northrup, M.D.*

- Faith is to the soul what a mainspring is to a watch.

- Genuine faith is assuring, insuring, and enduring.

- Feed your faith and your doubts will starve to death. – *Debbie Macomber*

- Faith keeps the man who keeps his faith.

- Faith gives us the courage to face the present with confidence, and the future with expectancy.

- If your faith cannot move mountains, it ought to at least climb them.

- What is faith but to believe what you do not see?

- Faith is something like electricity, you can't see it, but you can see the light. – *Gregory Dickow*

- Living without faith is like driving in a fog. – *E. Meehan*

- Faith with works is a force. Faith without works is a farce.

- No one can live in doubt when he has prayed in faith.

- Faith helps us walk fearlessly, run confidently, and live victoriously. – *Hagee Ministries*

- I tell you the truth, if you have faith as small as a mustard seed, you can say to this mountain, Faith is a refusal to panic. – *D. Martyn Lloyd-Jones*

- The object of your faith must be Christ. Not faith in ritual, not faith in sacrifices, not faith in morals, not faith in yourself — not faith in anything but Christ. – *Billy Graham*

- Everything that we see is a shadow cast by that which we do not see. – *Martin Luther King Jr.*

- Sorrow looks back, worry looks around and faith looks up. – *Anonymous*

- Now faith is the substance of things hoped for, the evidence of things not seen. – *Hebrews 11:1 KJV*

FAME

- If you think you are important, just remember that a lot of famous men of a century ago have weeds growing over their graves today.

- Money, achievement, fame, and success are important; but they are bought too dearly when acquired at the cost of health.

- No one ever traveled the road to fame on a free pass.

- The fame of great men ought always to be estimated by the means used to acquire it. – *François Duc de La Rochefoucauld*

FAMILY

- A family consists of a husband who gets an idea, the kids who say it can't be done, and the wife who does it.

- Keeping peace in the family requires patience, love, understanding, and at least two television sets.

- Marry and have children, and then find mates for them and have many grandchildren. Multiply! Don't dwindle away! – *Jeremiah 29:6*

- When does the family start? It starts with a young man falling in love with a girl. No superior alternative has yet been found. – *Winston Churchill*

- Men have sight; women insight. – *Victor Hugo*

- A grandmother is a person with too much wisdom to let that stop her from making a fool of herself over grandchildren. – *Phil Moss*

- The most wonderful thing ever made by man is a living for his family.

FAULTS

- A fault which humbles a man is of more use to him than a good action which puffs him up. – *Woodrow Wilson*

- All a bachelor has to do to discover his hidden faults is to get married.

- Each one of us finds in others the very faults others find in us.

- Human nature seems to endow every man with the ability to size up everybody but himself. – *John Maxwell*

- Justifying a fault doubles it. – *French Proverb*

- People will overlook the faults of anyone who is kind.

- Pride hides a man's fault to himself and magnifies them to everyone else.

- The man who thinks he has no faults has at least one.

- The worst fault of some people is telling other about theirs.

- To be swift to discuss the faults and follies of others does not necessarily imply that we are superior.

- You can shut your eyes to your own faults, but the neighbors always refuse to cooperate.

FEAR

- Courage is being the only one who knows you're afraid. – *Franklin P. Jones*

- Courage is not the absence of fear, but the conquest of it. – *Nelson Mandela*

- Don't let the future scare you — it's just as shaky as you are.

- Fear falls before the fortress of faith. – *Hagee Ministries*

- Fear is the tax that conscience pays to guilt. – *George Sewell*

- Fear of criticism is the kiss of death in the courtship of achievement.

- Fear of failure is the father of failure.

- Fear of the future is a waste of the present.

- Fear tends to produce the thing that it's afraid of.

- He who is afraid of doing too much always does too little.

- If you fear people will know it, don't do it.

- Many people are so filled with fear that they go through life running from something that isn't after them.

- Remember, you are your own doctor when it comes to curing cold feet.

- The greatest mistake you can make in this life is to be constantly fearful you will make one.

- The highway of fear is the shortest route to defeat.

- The one thing that is worse than a quitter is the man who is afraid to begin. – *Suzanne Woods Fisher*

- There is nothing so fearful as fear itself.

- Those who fear the future are likely to fumble the present. – *Amish Proverb*

- When you can think of yesterday without regret, and of tomorrow without fear, you are well on the road to success. – *Richard Denny*

Feelings

- Until today, you may not have understood that harboring feelings create tension in a relationship, and that what you feel is an important step toward healing yourself and another.

- Just for today lovingly express your feelings in a way that honors yourself and others. – *Iyanla Vanzant*

- Sometimes your best feelings are found in the words which you type and never send.

- Do unto others as you would like them to do unto you. – *Luke 6:31*

Fight

- Financial freedom comes when you take care of the people and the places around you, and you offer your services to God. – *Suze Orman*

- First be the best, then best the first.
  – *T Statement*

- ❦ Avoiding a fight is a mark of honor; only fools insist on quarreling. – *Proverbs 20:3*

- ❦ Don't pick a fight without reason, when no one has done you harm. – *Proverbs 3:30*

- ❦ Evil wins when the good doesn't fight.

FINANCE

- ❦ Your financial life is like a garden. If you tend a garden carefully- nourishing the flowers, pruning and weeding- it's going to be a lot more beautiful than if you simply water it halfheartedly now and then. – *Suze Orman*

- ❦ When it comes to every financial decision you'll make for the rest of your life, you'll choose correctly if you go with your first instinctual response. The answer will always be the right one for you, the one that will empower you to make money for yourself. – *Suze Orman*

- ❦ Spend not; want not.

Flattery

- Conscience is the only mirror that doesn't flatter.

- Flattery is like chewing gum. Enjoy it but don't swallow. – *Henry Ward*

- Insincere praise is worse than no praise at all.

Focus

- Take your focus off of how others see you. Cease being obsessed with the need to impress your friends and your foes. Keep your concern on the vision you see in the mirror. Don't allow the approval of others to obstruct your view of you. – *Tavis Smiley*

- Take your focus off of how others see you. Cease being upset us with the need to impress your friends and your photos. Keep your concern on the vision you see in the mirror. Don't allow the approval of others to obstruct your view of you. – *Tavis Smiley*

- When you have nothing left but God, then for the first time you become aware that God is enough. – *Maude Royden*

- I do not focus on who cares about me but on who I care about.

- I make each and every person with whom I communicate whether by phone, in person, in writing, or over the internet feel as if they are the focus of my world, at least for the duration of our interaction.

- I do not dwell on the past that I cannot change.

- Today, I am focusing on all the joy, kindness, and generosity there is within me and in the world.

FOOD

- Health rule: Eat like a king for breakfast, a prince for lunch, and a pauper for dinner. – *Adele Davis*

- A fool and his money are soon parted. The rest of us wait until we reach the supermarket.

- It's hard to keep a man's love with cold food.

꘍ Our greatest need at the present time is a cheap substitute for food.

Foolishness

꘍ Fools have no interest in understanding; they only want to air their own opinions. – *Proverbs 18:2*

꘍ Foolish children bring grief to their father and bitterness to the one who gave them birth. – *Proverbs 17:25*

꘍ The mouths of fools are their ruin; they trap themselves with their lips. – *Proverbs 18:7*

꘍ Every person, in their life has either done, or is doing or will do something foolish. – *TV Channel*

Forgiveness

꘍ Men with clenched fists cannot shake hands.

꘍ The supreme act of forgiveness is when you can forgive yourself for all the sounds you've created in your life. Forgives is an act of self-love. When you forgive yourself, self-acceptance begins and self-love grows. – *Don Miguel Ruiz*

- Forgive one person today. Open your heart to that person, and release unnecessary suffering from the past. Feel the peace that follows from this simple act. – *Caroline Myss and Peter Occhiogrosso*

- Forgive your parents, forgive your siblings, forgive your mate, forgive your friends, and forgive your enemies. Above all, forgive yourself. – *Tavis Smiley*

- Forgiveness is the most powerful thing you can do for yourself on the spiritual path. If you can't learn to forgive, you can forget about getting to higher levels of awareness. – *Dr. Wayne W. Dyer*

- There's no statute of limitations on forgiveness. In the presence or absence of explanation, forgive yourself and forgive others. – *Keith D. Harrell*

- When you recognize that your emotions, as well as others', can be capricious at times, you are better able to forgive and forget. – *Deepak Chopra. M.D*

- Two marks of a Christian: giving and forgiving.

- We should forgive and then forget what we have forgiven.

- We are like beasts when we kill. We are like men when we judge. We are like God when we forgive. – *William Arthur Ward*

- Forgiveness is the perfume that the trampled flower casts upon the heel that crushed it.

- It is far better to forgive and forget than to hate and remember.

- It isn't necessary to put a marker at the grave when we forgive and bury the hatchet.

- Forgiveness is the key that unlocks the door of resentment and the handcuffs of hate. It is a power that breaks the chains of bitterness and the shackles of selfishness. – *Corrie Ten Boom*

- The kindest people are those who forgive and forget.

- I believe that you must forgive whenever possible, but sometimes there are certain things or people you cannot forgive, no matter how hard you try. This is when you must give it to God for God is greater than you are and can take care of whatever you can't. – *Sylvia Browne*

FORTUNE

- ❦ I count what I have to be fortunate about and dwell on my good fortune.

- ❦ Fortune falls but once.

- ❦ Success is the good fortune that comes from aspiration, desperation, perspiration and inspiration. – *Evan Esar*

FRANKNESS

- ❦ Frankness doesn't require being brutally so.

- ❦ A man who says what he thinks is courageous, but friendless.

- ❦ People who say what they think would not be so bad if they thought.

Freedom

- Freedom is a package deal — with it comes responsibilities and consequences.

- Freedom is not the right to do as you please, but the liberty to do as you should. – *Ralph Waldo Emerson*

- Freedom is like the air we breathe; we don't miss it until we're deprived of it.

- Freedom ends when it begins to deprive another of his freedom.

- Freedom is not only the right to use your judgement, but the obligation to live with the consequences.

- Freedom is the right all people have to be as happy as they can.

- Freedom is indivisible. It is for all or none.

- No one but us can free our minds. – *Bob Marley*

- As a general rule, the freedom of any people can be judged by the volume of their laughter. – *Anupam Kher*

- Freedom is the sure possession of those alone who have the courage to defend it. – *Pericles*

FRIENDS

- The more arguments you win, the fewer friends you'll have.

- As long as your conscience is your friend, never mind about your enemies.

- A friend will see you through after others see you are through.

- Seldom visits make best friends. – *Dr. Voletta Williams*

- A friend that isn't in need is a friend indeed.

- Friends are like a priceless treasure; he who has none is a social pauper.

- Friends last longer the less they are used.

- A real friend warms you by his presence, trusts you with his secrets, and remembers you in his prayers.

- A good friend is one who can tell you all his problems — but doesn't.

- A true friend thinks of you when all others are thinking of themselves.

- A friend is one who is there to care.

- A real friend is one who walks in when the rest of the world walks out. – *Walter Winchell*

- A friend is a person who knocks before he enters, not after he has taken his departure.

- A real friend will tell you your faults and follies in times of prosperity, and assist you with his hand and heart in times of adversity.

- Some friends are like your shadow — you see them only when the sun shines. – *Michael Jackson*

- A task worth doing and friends worth having make life worthwhile.

- Your popularity will depend on *how* you treat your friends — and how often!

- A man's reputation is a blend of what his friends, enemies, and acquaintances say behind his back.

- When a man has climbed high on the ladder of success, quite often some of his friends begin to shake the ladder.

- It is extremely difficult for a man who loses his temper to hold his friends.

FRIENDSHIP

- An offended friend is harder to win back than a fortified city. Arguments separate friends like a gate locked with bars. – *Proverbs 18:19*

- Birds of the same feather flock together. – *English Proverb*

- Do not use a hatchet to remove a fly from, your friend's forehead. – *Chinese Proverb*

- Friends are lost by calling often and calling seldom. – *Scottish Proverb*

- Friendship is a living thing that lasts only as long as it is nourished with kindness, sympathy, and understanding. – *Mary Lou Retton*

- Genuine friendship is like sound health; its value is seldom known until it is lost.

- If one falls down, his friend can help him up. But pity the man who falls and has no one to help him up! – *Ecclesiastes 4:10*

- It takes a long time to grow an old friend. – *John Leonard*

- Many seek favors from a ruler; everyone is the friend of a person who gives gifts! – *Proverbs 19:6*

- Never abandon a friend — either yours or your father's. – *Proverbs 27:10*

- Show me your friends and I will show you your future.

- Tell me with whom you go and I will tell you what you are. A man is known by the company he keeps.

- The best mirror is an old friend. – *George Herbert*

- There are "friends" who destroy each other, but a real friend sticks closer than a brother. – *Proverbs 18:24*

- True friends are like diamonds, precious but rare while false friends are like autumn leaves found everywhere. – *Victor Anyaso*

- Wealth makes many "friends;" poverty drives them all away. – *Proverbs 19:4*

- When you choose your friends, make sure that they are assets and not liabilities.

- Wise is the man who fortifies his life with friendships. – *Colin Powell*

FRUITS

- Good thoughts bear good fruit, bad thoughts bear bad fruit — and man is his own Gardner. – *James Allen*

- … In order to live a happy life and the only thing we need is moral goodness. – *Cicero, Discussions at Tusculum.*

- A fruit doesn't fall to far from the tree.

FUTURE

- It's better to look where you're going than to see where you've been.

- Faith gives us the courage to face the present with confidence and the future with expectancy.

- Those who fear the future are likely to fumble the present. – *Amish Proverb*

- Hats off to the past, coats off to the future. – *Clare Booth Luce*

- When all is lost, the future still remains. – *Christian Nestell Bovee*

- Those who remember the past with a clear conscience need to have no fear of the future.

- No one can walk backward into the future. – *Joseph Hergesheimer*

- Memories are the key not to the past, but to the future. – *Corrie ten Boom*

- Anticipating is even more fun than recollection. – *Malcolm S. Forbes*

- Nobody gets to live life backward. Look ahead — that's where your future lies. – *Ann Landers*

- Far away is far away only if you don't go there. – *Anonymous*

- The future holds something in store for the individual who keeps faith in it.

- The future will be different if we make the present different. – *Peter Maurin*

- The future frightens only those who prefer living in the past.

- More people worry about the future than prepare for it.

- A pessimist burns his bridges before he gets to them. – *Sidney Ascher*

- One way to cover up a bad past is to build a big future over it.

- The best is yet to be. – *Robert Browning*

- You may not have been responsible for your heritage, but you are responsible for your future.

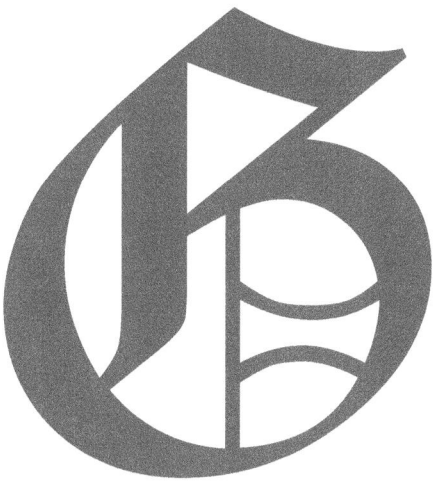

Genealogies

- Noble and common blood is of the same color. – *German Proverb*

- Parents who wonder where the younger generation is going should remember where it came from. – *Sam Ewing*

- Before more people start boasting about their family tree, they usually do a good pruning job. – *O.A. Battista*

Generosity

- Feel for others — in your pocket! – *Charles H. Spurgeon*

- The open hand holds more friends than the closed fist.

- Generosity will always leave a more pleasant memory than stinginess.

- He who gives only when he is asked has waited too long.

- Wisdom enables one to be thrifty without being stingy, and generous without being wasteful.

- A genius shoots at something no one else sees — and hits it!

- True generosity lies not in how much money you have, but whether the money you have coming in and going out passes through your heart back out into the world. – *Suze Orman*

- Make others the focal point. Give generously, listen intently, praise freely, and love unceasingly. Take the spotlight off yourself and shine it on others. – *Tavis Smiley*

- To handle yourself, use your head; to handle others, use your heart. – *Eleanor Roosevelt (Feb 2019)*

- Your generosity toward others is key to your positive experiences in the world. Know that there's enough room for everyone to be passionate, creative, and successful. In fact, there's more than enough room for everyone; there's need for everyone. – *Marianne Williamson*

- Don't visit your neighbors too often, or you will wear out your welcome. – *Proverbs 25:17*

- Give freely and become more wealthy; be stingy and lose everything. – *Proverbs 11:24*

- I am focusing on what I can give to others.

- Whoever gives to the poor will lack nothing, but those who close their eyes to poverty will be cursed. – *Proverbs 28:27*

- The generous will prosper; those who refresh others will themselves be refreshed. – *Proverbs 11:25*

- I am happy giving to others.

Genius

- Men of genius are admired; men of wealth are envied; men of power are feared; but only men of character are trusted. – *Alfred Adler*

- Genius is nothing more than inflamed enthusiasm.

- Genius is the ability to reduce the complicated to the simple.

- Genius is 1 percent inspiration and 99 percent perspiration. – *Thomas Edison*

- Often GENIUS is just another way of spelling perseverance.

- So few people think. When we find one who really does, we call him a genius.

GENTLENESS

- Nothing is so strong as gentleness and nothing is so gentle as real strength. – *Saint Francis de Sales*

- Gentle words are a tree of life; a deceitful tongue crushes the spirit. – *Proverbs 15:4*

- Say little. But when you speak, utter gentle words that touch the heart. Be truthful. Express kindness. Abstain from vanity. This is the Way. – *Daniel Levin*

GIFTS

- The greatest gift we can bestow on others is a good example. – *Thomas Morell*

- A practical gift is one you can afford.

- If we bestow a gift or a favor and expect a return for it, it's not a gift but a trade.

- Giving money month-in, month-out is a way of saying thank you to the world and also a way of saying please. A pure charitable gift will always be returned — many times over. – *Suze Orman.*

- Sharing your gifts with the world.

- Giving a gift can open doors; it gives access to important people! – *Proverbs 18:16*

- You could never repay all you've been given by the creator. Except gifts. Live and share them. – *Anne Wilson Schaef*

GIVING

- Advice is the one thing which is *"more blessed to give than to receive."*

- Charity begins at home, and generally dies from lack of outdoor exercise.

- Blessed are those who can give without remembering, and receive without forgetting. – *Elizabeth Bibesco*

- Feel for others — in your pocket. – *Charles H. Spurgeon*

- Don't give 'til it hurts — give 'til it feels good. – *Dennis Kimbro*

- Give not from the top of your purse, but from the bottom of your heart.

- *"It is more blessed to give than to receive"* is often quoted but seldom practiced.

- We make a living by what we get, but we make a life by what we give. – *Winston Churchill*

- Giving until it hurts is not a true measure of generosity. Some are easier hurt than others.

- What you give lives!

- You can give without loving, but you can't love without giving. – *Amy Carmichael*

- The manner of giving is worth more than the gift. – *Pierre Corneille*

- Giving is the thermometer of our love.

- The world is composed of givers and takers. The takers may eat better but the givers sleep better. – *Gaur Gopal Das*

GOALS

- Some fellows dream of worthy accomplishments, while others stay awake and do them.

- Having a great aim in life is important. So is knowing when to pull the trigger.

- It's better to aim at a good thing and miss it than to aim at a bad thing and hit it.

- There's no sense aiming for a goal with no arrow in your bow.

- Following the path of least resistance is what makes rivers and men crooked.

- You are never too old to set another goal or dream a new dream. – *C.S. Lewis*

- ❦ Set a goal, write it down, and release the outcome. Small steps make a big difference. – *Cheryl Richardson*

- ❦ People with goals succeed because they know where they are going. – *Earl Nightingale*

- ❦ The greatest thing in this world is not so much where we are, but in what direction we are moving.

- ❦ Having a goal makes me happy, so I have a goal for today.

- ❦ I am making happiness a goal and a priority, and I am working on the goal.

- ❦ Goals are tools for focusing on your life and for inspiring you to take action. Today, determine the worth of your goals… because everything you want may not actually be worth having. – *Keith D. Harrell*

Godliness

- ❦ The wicked are trapped by their own words, but the godly escape such trouble. – *Proverbs 12:13*

- ❧ Don't wait in ambush at home of the godly, and don't raid the house where the godly live. – *Proverbs 24:15*

- ❧ The godly may trip seven times, but they will get up again. But one disaster is enough to overthrow the wicked. – *Proverbs 24:16*

- ❧ Evil people get rich for the moment, but the reward of the godly will last. – *Proverbs 11:18*

- ❧ Godly people find life; evil people find death. – *Proverbs 11:19*

- ❧ When the godly are in authority, the people rejoice. But when the wicked are in power they groan. – *Proverbs 29:2*

- ❧ Evil people will surely be punished, but the children of the godly will go free. – *Proverbs 11:21*

- ❧ No harm comes to the godly, but the wicked have their fill of trouble. – *Proverbs 12:21*

- ❧ The godly can look forward to a reward, while the wicked can expect only judgment. – *Proverbs 11:23*

- ❧ Wickedness never brings stability, but the godly have deep roots. – *Proverbs 12:3*

- The plans of the godly are just; the advice of the wicked is treacherous. – *Proverbs 12:5*

- The words of the wicked are like a numerous ambush, but the words of the godly save lives. – *Proverbs 12:6*

- The wicked die and disappear, but the family of the godly stands firm. – *Proverbs 12:7*

- Better to have little, with godliness, than to be rich and dishonest. – *Proverbs 16:8*

- The godly are rescued from troubles, and it falls on the wicked instead.

- The godliness of good people rescues them; the ambition of treacherous people traps them. – *Proverbs 11:6*

- Cleanliness may be next to godliness, but in childhood it's next to impossible.

Goodness

- The man who cannot be angry at evil usually lacks enthusiasm for good. – *Dr. David Seamands*

- ❦ Few people make a deliberate choice between good and evil; the choice is between what we want to do and what we ought to do.

- ❦ Between two evils, choose neither; between two goods, choose both. – *Tryon Edwards*

- ❦ The best way to escape evil is to pursue good.

- ❦ We do more good by being good than in any other way.

- ❦ Do not be simply good — be good for something. – *Henry David Thoreau*

- ❦ Goodness consists not so much in the outward things we do, but in the inward things we are. – *Edwin Hubbell Chapin*

- ❦ Greatness is not found in possessions, power, position, or prestige. It is discovered in goodness, humility, service, and character.

GRACE

- ❦ Grace is but glory begun, and glory is but grace perfected. – *Jonathan Edwards*

- There is nothing sadder or glorious than GENERATIONS changing hands. – *John Cougar Mellencamp*

- Wherever life plants you, bloom with grace.

Gratitude

- If you can't be content with what you have received, be thankful for what you have escaped. – *Izaak Walton*

- Our favorite attitude should be gratitude.

- Debts of gratitude are the most difficult to collect.

- There is a sense in which no gift is ours till we have thanked the giver.

- Gratitude is the rarest of all virtues, and yet we invariably expect it.

- Express gratitude generously and sincerely; receive gratitude humbly and graciously; expect gratitude rarely, if ever.

- Be grateful for what you have, not regretful for what you haven't.

- Gratitude is not only the greatest of virtues, but the parent of all the others. – *Marcus Tullius Cicero*

- Gratitude is the most exquisite form of courtesy. – *Jacques Maritain*

- Do not burn the bridge behind your back.

- I have gratitude for those who have given to me in any and all ways.

- There are two kinds of people in the world: those who pull you up and those who pull you down. Identify the people who pull you up and show them an attitude of gratitude. – *Keith D. Harrell*

GREATNESS

- The measure of a truly great man is the courtesy with which he treats lesser men.

- Greatness lies not in being strong, but in the right use of strength. – *Henry Ward Beecher*

- Greatness is not found in possessions, power, position, or prestige. It is discovered in goodness, humility, service, and character. – *William Arthur Ward*

- A great man is one who can have power and not abuse it. – *Henry Latham Dohertty*

- There is not true greatness where simplicity, goodness, and truth are absent.

- Great men, like the tallest mountain, retain their majesty and stability during the most severe storm.

- A man must be big enough to admit his mistakes, smart enough to profit from them, and strong enough to correct them. – *John C. Maxwell*

- Every great person first learned how to obey, whom to obey, and when to obey. – *William Arthur Ward*

- Great things are done by a series of small things brought together. – *Vincent Van Gogh*

- Patience is the companion of wisdom. – *Saint Augustine*

- Great principles do not need men and women as much as men and women need great principles.

GROWTH

- Some people grow up and still remain both juvenile and delinquent.

- Knowledge has to be improved, challenged, and increased constantly or it vanishes.

- Some men grow; others just swell.

- Try different ventures and experiences as a way to grow and learn. – *Dorian Virtue. Ph.D.*

- Never too old to learn new.

- Unless you try to do something beyond what you have already mastered, you will never grow.

- Meanwhile, the church had peace throughout Judea, Galilee, and Samaria, and grew in strength and numbers. The believers learned how to walk in the fear of the Lord and in the comfort of the Holy Spirit. – *Acts 9:31*

- I may be old but I haven't stopped growing! – *Oliver Wendell Holmes, Jr.*

Guidance

- Keep your face to the sunshine and you cannot see a shadow. – *Helen Keller*

- She will guide you down delightful paths; all her ways are satisfying. – *Proverbs 3:17-18*

- Oh virgin mother, lady of good counsel, sweetest picture artists ever drew, in all my doubts I fly to thee for guidance. Oh mother tell me what I am to do. – *O Virgin Mother (Lady of Good Counsel), A Marian Song*

- The great thing in the world is not so much where we are, but in what direction we are moving. – *Oliver Wendell Holmes*

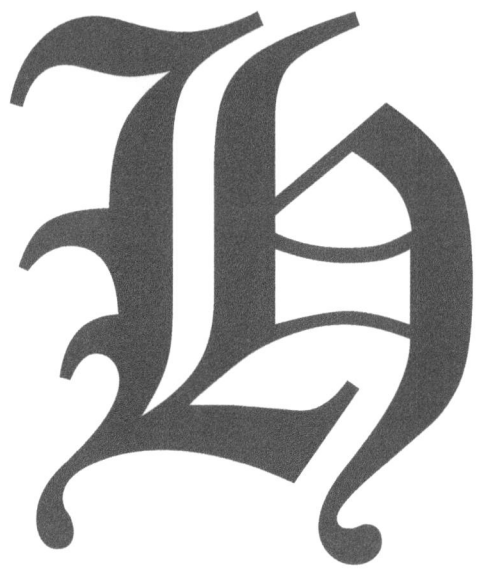

HABITS

- A habit is something a fellow hardly notices until it's too strong to break.

- Form good habits; they're as hard to break as bad ones.

- It's easier to form good habits than reform bad ones.

- Habits are like a soft bed — easy to get into but hard to get out of.

- Marriage is a case of two people agreeing to change each other's habits.

HAPPINESS

- A man has happiness in the palm of his hands if he can fill his days with real work and his nights with real rest.

- All we are guaranteed is the pursuit of happiness. You have to catch up with it yourself.

- For true happiness, look within yourself. It's difficult to be happy if you rely on outside sources. – *Keith D Harrell*

- Happiness does not come from what you have, but from what you are.

- Happiness is a by-product of achievement.

- Happiness is a healthy mental attitude, a grateful spirit, a clear conscience, and a heart full of love.

- Happiness is getting something you wanted but didn't expect.

- Happiness is not something you have in your hands; it is something you carry in your heart.

- Happiness is the result of being too busy to be miserable.

- Happiness will never come to those who fail to appreciate what they already have.

- He who forgets the language of gratitude can never be on speaking terms with happiness.

- If you cannot find happiness along the way, you will not find it at the end of the road.

- It isn't your position that makes you happy or unhappy. It's your disposition.

- One does not find happiness in marriage, but takes happiness into marriage.

- People whose main concern is their own happiness seldom find it.

- Some pursue happiness — others create it.

- The roots of happiness grow deepest in the soil of service.

- The secret of success and happiness lies not in doing what you like, but in liking what you do.

- Those who bring sunshine to the lives of others cannot keep it from themselves. – *James Barnee*

- To love others makes us happy; to love ourselves makes us lonely.

Harmony

- Happiness is not a matter of intensity but of balance and order and rhythm and harmony. – *Thomas Merton*

- Harmony is a beautiful balance between mind, body and soul measured in tender peaceful moments.

- Harmony makes small things grow, lack of it makes small things decay.

- Truth is inner harmony.

HATRED

- It is far better to forgive and forget than to hate and remember.

- Forgiveness saves the expense of anger, the high cost of hatred, and the waste of energy. – *Hannah More*

- Forgiveness is the key that unlocks the door of resentment and the handcuffs of hate. It is a power that breaks the chains of bitterness and the shackles of selfishness.

- Hatred is a boomerang which is sure to hit you harder than the one at whom you throw it.

- Hate is a luxury no one can afford.

- If you want to be miserable, hate somebody.

- Hatred is cancer of the intellect.

- There are many roads to hate, but envy is one of the shortest of them all.

- Hate pollutes the mind.

- The sunlight of love will kill all the germs of jealousy and hate.

- Hiding hatred makes you a liar; slandering others makes you a fool.

Healing

- I treated him, God cured him. – *Ambroise Pare*

- God heals, and the doctor takes the fee. – *Benjamin Franklin*

- What wound have you left unhealed? Are you willing to begin healing today?

- An unhealed wound drains you of the very energy needed to live beyond the wound. – *Iyanla Vanzant*

- Healing takes courage, and we all have courage, even if we have to dig a little to find it.

Health

- A lot of people lose their health trying to become wealthy, and then lose their wealth trying to get back their health.

- Many people suffer poor health, not because of what they eat, but form what is eating them.

- Money, achievement, fame, and success are important, but they are bought too dearly when acquired at the cost of health.

- The best health insurance is moderation.

- The human body, with proper care, will last a lifetime.

- Our health always seems much more valuable after we lose it.

- Health is the thing that makes you feel that *now* is the best time of the year.

- Those who ignore health in the pursuit of wealth usually wind up losing both.

- Anybody who thinks money is everything has never been sick.

- A good wife and good health are a man's best wealth.

- A healthy mind in a healthy body; a healthy voice in a healthy body.

- The ground work of all happiness is health. – *Leigh Hunt*

- The ground work to all happiness is health. – *Leigh Hunt, Walgreens Pharmacy*

- A healthy mind in a healthy body; a healthy voice in a healthy body.

- Keep the health and heaven will come.

- The ground work of all happiness is health. – *Leigh Hunt*

- A healthy mind in a healthy body is a healthy voice in a healthy body.

HEART

- Two things are bad for the heart — running upstairs and running down people.

- A small gift will do if your heart is big enough.

- Give not from the top of your purse, but from the bottom of your heart.

- The door to the human heart can be opened only from the inside.

- There is no better exercise for the heart than reaching down and lifting people up.

- In judging others it's always wise to see with the heart as well as with the eyes.

- Kindness is the insignia of a loving heart.

- The most lonely place in the world is the human heart when love is absent.

- Peace is not made in documents, but in the hearts of men.

- Heads, hearts, and hands could settle the world's problems better than arms.

- A smile is the lighting system of the face and the heating system of the heart.

- If there is a smile in your heart, your face will show it.

- The smile that lights the face will also warm the heart.
- Sympathy is the result of thinking with your heart.
- Tolerance is seeing things with your heart instead of your eyes.

HELP

- It is one of the most compensations of this life that no man can sincerely trying to help anther without helping himself. – *Ralph Waldo Emerson*
- Ask for help. Receiving is an act of generosity. – *Cheryl Richardson*
- If you can help your neighbor now, don't say, *"Come back tomorrow, and then I'll help you."*
- I seek out professional help for my depression without shame if I need outside help.
- Until today, you may have been feeling overwhelmed by trying to do everything on your own. Just for today, ask God to help you ease some of your burdens. – *Iyanla Vanzant*

Helpfulness

- True charity is helping those you have every reason to believe would not help you.

- To feel sorry for the needy is not the mark of a Christian — to help them is.

- It's nice to know that when you help someone up a hill you are a little nearer the top yourself.

- The open hand holds more friends than the closed fist.

History

- He who does not remember the past is condemned to forget where he parked.

- History is nothing more than the art of reconciling fact with fiction.

- History is simply a record of man's intelligence — or lack of it.

- History is to a nation what memory is to the individual.

- History repeats itself — and that's one of the things wrong with history.

- History reveals that wars create more problems than they solve.

- Leaders go down in history. Some farther down than others.

- Those who cannot remember the past are condemned to repeat it. – *George Santayana*

- You can clutch the past so tightly to your chest that it leaves your arms too full to embrace the present. – *Jan Glidewell*

Hoarding

- Circulate dormant possessions. Don't hang on to items you aren't using just because you spent good money on them, because if you need them again, they will probably find their way back to you. – *Julie Morgenstern*

❧ If you have trouble letting go of unused possessions, then adopt a charity or give them to a friend! It's easier to part with items if they're going to an organization or person you care about. – *Julie Morgenstern*

❧ Improve your quality of life. Give yourself access to the things you use and love by getting rid of the stuff you don't. – *Julie Morgenstern*

HOME

❧ A person who strays from home is like a bird that strays from its nest.

❧ A house without love may be a castle or a palace, but it is not a home … – *Sam Ewing*

❧ By wisdom a house is built, and through understanding it is established; through knowledge its rooms are filled with rare and beautiful treasures. – *Proverbs 24:3-4*

Honesty

- The most important person to be honest with is yourself.

- It takes a mighty honest man to tell the difference between when he's tired and when he's just plain lazy.

- You are your word. Say what you will do, and do what you say. Never call your word into questions with lies, deceit, or misrepresentation. Create credibility by honoring your word. – *Tavis Smiley*

- It pays more than it costs to be honest.

- Honesty gives a person strength but not always popularity.

- All men are honest — until they are faced with a situation tempting enough to make them dishonest.

- An honest man alters his ideas to fit the truth, and a dishonest man alters the truth to fit his ideas.

- Honesty is a question of right and wrong, not a matter of policy.

- live your life so that your autograph will be wanted instead of your fingerprints.

- The person who is straightforward and honest doesn't have to worry about a faulty memory.

- People who wink at the wrong cause trouble, but a bold reproof promoted peace.

- The king is pleased with words from righteous lips; he loves those who speak honestly.

- An honest witness tells the truth; a false witness tells lies.

- Get the truth and never sell it; also get wisdom, discipline, and good judgement.

- An honest answer is like a kiss of friendship.

- Don't cheat your neighbor by moving the ancient boundary markers set up by previous generations.

- Honesty guides good people; dishonesty treacherous people.

- An honest witness does not lie; a false witness breathes lies.

- ❦ A clear conscience fears no accusation.

- ❦ Good name in man and woman dear my lord is the immediate treasure of our souls. He who steals my purse steals trash. It was mine, it is his and has been friends to thousands but he who robs me of my good name filches me of that which thou not enriches him but me poor indeed.

Honor

- ❦ The guilty walk a crooked path; the innocent travel a straight road.

- ❦ I look at what is positive and praiseworthy about those I love rather than to be critical.

- ❦ Honor may not win power, but it earns respect.

Hope

- ❦ Faith, hope, and charity — if we had more of the first two we'd need less of the last.

- There's more hope for a confessed sinner than a conceited saint.

- Hope sees the invisible, feels the intangible, and achieves the impossible.

- You can't live on hope alone, nor can you live without it.

- Hope is the anchor of the soul, the stimulus to action, and the incentive to achievement.

- Hope is faith holding out its hand in the dark.

- Ideals may be beyond our reach but never beyond our fondest hopes.

- Hope for the best, and be ready for the worst.

- If it were not for hopes, the heart would break. – *Thomas Fuller*

- We must accept finite disappointment, but we must never lose infinite hope. – *Martin Luther King, Jr.*

- Some people grumble because rose has thorns. I am thankful that thorns have roses. – *Karr*

- It ain't over till it's over. – *Lawrence "Yogi" Berra*

- For this day, acknowledge the restoring power of hope. Direct that power to bless all that needs healing in your life, including your negative attitude and disappointments. – *Caroline Myss and Peter Ochiogrosso*

- One cannot change yesterday, but can only make the most of today, and look with hope toward tomorrow.

- Hope deferred makes the heart sick, but a dream fulfilled is a tree of life.

- The hopes of the godly result in happiness, but the expectations of the wicked come to nothing.

- When the wicked die, their hope dies with them, for they rely on their own feeble strength.

- For the despondent, every day brings trouble; for the happy heart, life is a continual feast.

Humanity

- We learn some things from prosperity, but we learn many more from adversity.

- An angry man is seldom reasonable; a reasonable man is seldom angry.

- Caution is what we call cowardice in others.

- By nature, all men are much alike, but by education they become different.

- An egotist is a man who talks so much about himself that he gives us no time to talk about ourselves.

- There are no great men except those who have rendered serve to mankind.

- Some pursue happiness — others create it.

- The plain fact is that human beings are happy only when they are striving for something worthwhile. What is it about human nature that makes it easier to break a commandment than a habit?

- Our five senses are incomplete without the sixth — a sense of humor.

- No law, however stringent, can make the idle industrious, the shiftless provident, or the drunkard sober.

- The weakness of man is the thing to be feared, not his strength.

- Most people make the mistake of looking too far ahead for things close by.

- It is almost impossible to smile on the outside without feeling better on the inside.

- Most people can resist everything but temptation.

- Think small and you'll remain small.

Humility

- It is when we forget ourselves that we do things that are most likely to be remembered.

- The fellow who does things that count doesn't usually stop to count them.

- Greatness is not found in possessions, power, position, or prestige. It is discovered in goodness, humility, service, and character.

- Humility is the ability to look properly shy when you tell people how wonderful you are.

- To be humble to superiors is duty; to equals, courtesy; to inferiors, nobility.

- Sincere humility attracts. Lack of humility subtracts. Artificial humility detracts.

- Stay humble or stumble.

- Humility is one of the qualities often left out of the "self-made" man.

- Humility and self-denial are always admired but seldom practiced.

- Don't brag about tomorrow, since you don't know what the day will bring.

- Let someone else praise you, not your own mouth—a stranger, not your own lips.

- Pride leads to disgrace, but with humility comes wisdom.

- Pride ends in humiliation, while humility brings honor.

- Power is dangerous unless you have humility.

- The sufficiency of my merit is to know that my merit is not sufficient. – *St. Augustine*

- The really tough thing about true humility is you can't brag about it. – *Gene Brown*

- Nothing is as hard to do gracefully as getting down off your high horse. – *Franklin P. Jones*

- Those who travel the high road of humility are not troubled by heavy traffic. – *Alan K. Simpson*

- Humility is a major component in being thankful, but being too humble leaves the soul in a state of feeling "not worthy". Be humble, but take pride in the fact that you have made it in life with God's grace. – *Sylvia Browne*

- Do not have your concert first and tune your instruments afterward. Begin the day with God. – *J. Hudson Taylor*

HUMOR

- Our five senses are incomplete without the sixth — a sense of humor.

- A well-developed sense of humor is the pole that adds balance to our steps as we walk the tightrope of life. – *William Arthur Ward*

- Humor is the lubricating oil of business. It prevents friction and wins good will.

- A sense of humor is a test of sanity.

Hypocrisy

- I cannot give you the formula for success, but I can give you the formula for failure — which is: Try to please everybody. – *Herbert Bayard Swope*

- Most people have seen worse things in private than they pretend to be shocked at in public. – *Edgar Watson Howe*

- A hypocrite is a person who preaches by the yard, but practices by the inch.

- A hypocrite never intends to be what he pretends to be.

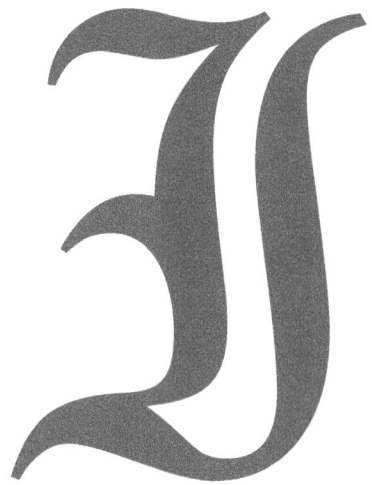

IDLENESS

- It pays to keep your feet on the ground, but keep them moving.

- No thoroughly occupied man has ever been known to be miserable.

- It's what you do when you have nothing to do that revels what you are.

- Few things are more dangerous to a person's character than having nothing to do and plenty of time in which to do it.

- When you don't want to do anything, one excuse is as good as another.

- The chief reward for idleness is poverty.

- The hardest job of all is trying to look busy when you're not.

- When an idler sees a job completed, he's sure he could have done it better.

- Idleness travels so slowly that poverty soon overtakes it.

- Idleness is the nest in which mischief lays its eggs.

- No one ever stumbled onto anything worthwhile sitting down.

- A little knowledge that acts is worth infinitely more than much knowledge that is idle.

- Never has a man who lived a life of ease left a name worth remembering.

IGNORANCE

- It is impossible to defeat an ignorant man in an argument.

- Discussion is an exchange of knowledge; argument is an exchange of ignorance.

- Many of the most firmly held beliefs are based solidly on ignorance.

- It's all right to be ignorant, but it's stupid to make a career out of it.

- Ignorance needs no introduction; it always makes itself known.

- There is nothing more terrifying than ignorance in action.

- It's harder to conceal ignorance than to acquire knowledge.

- Ignorance of law is no excuse, neither is the ignorance of the lawmakers.

- Knowledge may have its limits, but not so with ignorance.

- The only known cure for ignorance is education.

- Many a man is not suspected of being ignorant till he starts to talk.

- A little learning may be a dangerous thing — but it's still safer than total ignorance.

- Ignorance of the law is no excuse, but it's better than no alibi at all.

- It's better to know nothing than to know what isn't so.

- Ignorance of the law is no excuse, except for judges.

- A truly great leader is one who never allows his followers to discover that he is as ignorant as they are.

- If you wish to get along with people, pretend not to know whatever they tell you.

- Prejudice is essentially an outgrowth of ignorance.

- Silence is the best and surest way to hide ignorance.

- When Ignorance is bliss, it is folly to be wise.

IMAGINATION

- Imagination is what makes you think you're having a wonderful time when you are only spending money.

- Unlike an aircraft, your imagination can take flight day or night and in any kind of weather.

- Imagination is what makes the average man think he can run the business better than his boss.

- The imagination is the powerhouse that supplies the mysterious force which we call "inspiration."

- Stretch your imagination too far and it will snap back at you.

- When temptation knocks, imagination usually answers.

- Everything you can imagine is real. – *Pablo Picasso*

- Logic will get you from A to B. Imagination will take you everywhere. – *Albert Einstein.*

- The pessimist sees difficulty in every opportunity. The optimist sees the opportunity in every difficulty. – *Sir Winston Churchill*

- I appreciate philosopher Immanuel Kant's words: *"Happiness is not an Ideal of reason but of Imagination."*

Importance

- Valuing the differences between people is the essence of synergy. Truly effective people have the humility to recognize their own perceptual limitations and appreciate the resources available through interactions with others. – *Stephen R. Covey*

- I value each and every day and I try to make the most of it because I do not know what tomorrow will bring.
- I hold firm those values that I should never waver on.
- I am more than any material gifts that I get or give.

IMPROVEMENT

- People seldom improve when they have no model but themselves.
- People seldom improve when they have no model to copy but themselves.
- Nobody ever does his best; that's why we all have a good chance to do better.
- Each person has the chance to improve himself, but some just don't believe in taking chances.
- The largest room in the world is the room for improvement.

Independence

- If you want to achieve greatness, stop asking for permission.

- If you don't paddle your own canoe, you don't move.

- Choose to be your own person.

- We need to give from the perspective of empowering the recipient instead of making them dependent on us. – *Tony Elumelu*

- People take different roads seeking fulfillment and happiness. Just because they're not on your road doesn't mean they've gotten lost. – *H. Jackson Browne*

- My children are responsible for their own happiness.

Industry

- If there is no struggle, there is no progress. – *Frederick Douglass*

- The harder you work the luckier you get. – *Carl Player*

- If you love sleep, you will end in poverty. Keep your eyes open and they would be plenty to eat!

- A hard worker has plenty of food, but a person who chases fantasies has no sense.

- Wise words bring many benefits, and hard work brings rewards.

- Work hard and become a leader; be lazy and become a slave.

- Lazy people are soon poor; hard workers get rich.

- Lazy people want much but get little, but those who work hard will prosper.

- A wise youth harvests in the summer, but one who sleeps during the harvest is a disgrace.

INFERIORITY

- No one can make you feel inferior without your permission.

- No one can make you feel inferior without your consent.

- One who has an inferiority complex can never be really humble, but can only have false modesty or humility.

INFLUENCE

- Example is not the main thing in influencing others. It is the only thing.

- Please don't try to use your influence until you're sure you have it.

- It is impossible for you to influence others to live on a higher level than that on which you live yourself.

- Influence is something you *think* you have until you try to use it.

- Just one act of yours may turn the tide of another person's life.

INGENUITY

- A child can ask questions that a wise man cannot answer.

- Never tell people how to do things. Tell them what to do and they will surprise you with their ingenuity.

- Lots of ingenuity gets you through times with no money better than money gets you through times of no ingenuity.

- Innovation comes out of great human ingenuity and very personal passions.

INITIATIVE

- Taking the initiative doesn't mean being pushy, obnoxious or aggressive. It means creating an atmosphere where others can seize opportunities and solve problems in an increasingly reliant way. – *Stephen R. Covey*

- Initiative is doing the right thing without being told.

- One has to take initiative in life to achieve what he or she wants.

- The journey of a thousand miles begins with one step. – *Lao Tzu*

INSATIABILITY

- Much would gain more and lose all. – *Prof. Alex D. W. Acholonu*

- Your heart is not large enough to contain the blessings that God wants to give. He pours and pours until they literally flew over the edge and down on the table. The last thing you need to worry about is having enough. – *Max Lucado*

- Just as Death and Destruction are never satisfied, so human desire is never satisfied. – *Proverbs 27:20*

INSCRIPTION

- The pen is mightier than the sword.

- The faintest ink is better than the finest memory. – *Ronald Anderson*

- The say the test of literary power is whether a man can write an inscription.

INSISTENCE

- ꙮ The difference between winning and losing is most often not quitting. – *Walt Disney*

- ꙮ Patience produces rose.

- ꙮ A patient dog eats the fattest bone.

- ꙮ Direct action is, ultimately, the defiant insistence on acting as if one is free.

INSPIRATION

- ꙮ The most important thing is to try and inspire people so that they can be great in whatever they want to do. – *Kobe Bryant*

- ꙮ Beauty awakens the soul to act.

- ꙮ The words of the godly encourage many, but fools are destroyed by their lack of common sense.

Instructions

- Instruct the wise, and they will be even wiser. Teach the righteous, and they will learn even more.

- A word is enough for the wise.

- Assessment is today's means of modifying tomorrow's instruction.

Intelligence

- It is not the I.Q. but the *I will* that is important in education.

- Not all educated people are intelligent.

- Enthusiasm is a good engine, but it needs intelligence for a driver.

- Facts mean nothing unless they are rightly understood, rightly related, and rightly interpreted.

- Intelligent people are always ready to learn. Their ears are open for knowledge.

INTENTIONS

- Small deeds done are better than great deeds planned.

- The smallest good deed is better than the grandest intention.

- There are few people who are fast enough to keep up with their good intentions.

- Good intentions die unless they are executed.

- Make sure your intentions are not just pretentions.

- The kindness we resolve to show tomorrow cures no headaches today.

- No one can build a reputation on what he's going to do tomorrow.

- The prudent understand where they are going, but fools deceive themselves.

INTERACTION

- Create opportunities to interact one-on-one with your boss, your children, your spouse, your friends, and your employees. When you listen, you learn, which opens the door to create solutions and mutual trust. – *Stephen R. Covey*

- Use each interaction to be the best, most powerful version of yourself.

- Treat every interaction like the most important meeting of your career.

- All human interactions are opportunities either to learn or to teach.

INTEREST

- People rarely succeed at anything unless they have fun doing it.

- Always remember, someone's effort is a reflection of their interest in you.

- The true secrets of happiness lies in taking a genuine interest in all the details of daily life.

INVENTION

- The best way to predict the future is to invent it. – *Alan Kay*
- Necessity is the mother of invention.
- It is obvious that anything a scientist discovers or invents is based on previous discoveries and inventions.
- The greatest invention of mankind is the compound interest. – *Albert Einstein*

IRRESPONSIBILITY

- The wicked bluff their way through, but the virtuous think before they act.

- Responsibility finds a way. Irresponsibility makes excuses.

- It's better to go to a neighbor than to a brother who lives far away.

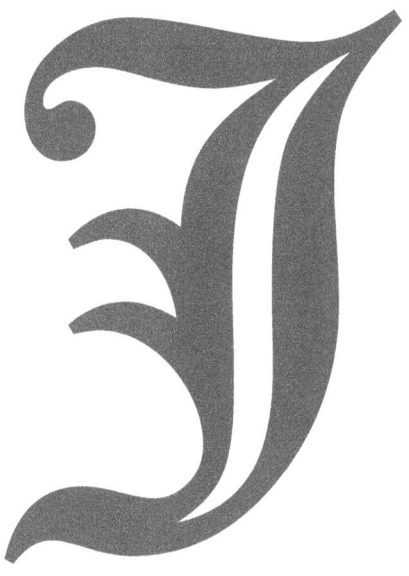

Jealousy

- Thieves are jealous of each other's loot, but the godly are well rooted and bear own fruit.

- Anger is cruel, and wrath is like a flood, but jealousy is even more dangerous.

- They are not jealous of what you have. They are jealous of what they can't have.

Journey

- Everywhere is walking distance if you have the time. – *Steven Wright*

- If all difficulties were known at the outset of a long journey, most of us would never start out at all. – *William Arthur Ward*

- Far away is far away only if you don't go there. – *Anonymous*

- There are no shortcuts to any place worth going. – *Bevrly Sills*

- Do not follow where the path may lead… Go instead where there is no path and leave a trail. Well done is better than well said. – *Ben Franklin*

- Only those who will risk going too far can possibly find out how far one can go. – *T.S. Eliot*

- The journey of a thousand miles starts with a single step. – *Chinese Proverb*

- Create new paths to follow.

- Everyone journeys through character as well as through time. The person one becomes depends on the person one has been. – *Benjamin Franklin*

JOY

- Selfishly seek joy, because your joy is the greatest gift you can give to anyone. Unless you are in your joy, you have nothing to give anyway. – *Abraham Hicks*

- A cheerful look brings joy to the heart; good news makes for good health.

- I dwell on the joy of my life.

- I define myself by joy and cheer.

- Laughter is the shortest distance between two people. *– Victor Borge*

- No matter how dull, or how mean, or how wise a man is, he feels that happiness is his indisputable right. *– Helen Keller*

- Laughter is a tranquilizer with no side effects. *– Arnold H. Glasow*

- Most people are about as happy as they make up their minds to be. *– Abraham Lincoln*

- Happiness is good health and a bad memory. *– Ingrid Bergman*

- I rejoice in the simple things of life.

JUDGEMENT

- Flipping a coin can end arguments; it settles disputes between powerful opponents.

- Leave your simple ways behind, and begin to live. Learn to use good judgment.

- Punishment is justice for the unjust. – *St. Augustine*

- Make no judgements where you have no compassion. – *Anne McCaffrey*

- Out of the frying-pan into the fire. – *Tertullian*

JUSTICE

- A king detests wrongdoing, for his rule is built on justice.

- Justice is a joy to the godly, but it terrifies evildoers.

- The first to speak in court sounds right, until the cross-examination begins.

- It is not right to acquit the guilty or deny justice to the innocent.

- Every day is for the thief, and one day is for the owner of the house.

- If you only hear one side of the story, you have no understanding at all. – *Chinua Achebe.*

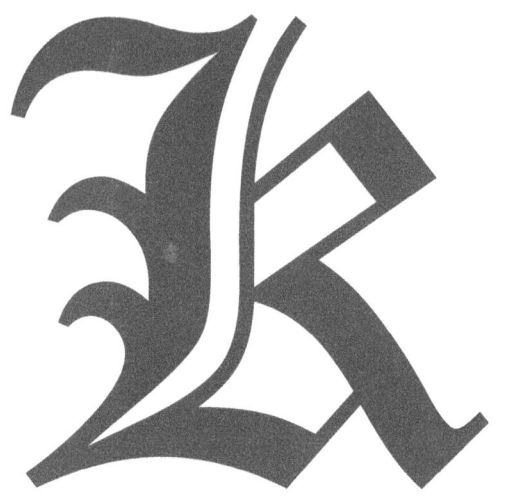

Kindness

- Friendship is a living thing that lasts only as long as it is nourished with kindness, sympathy, and understanding.

- The person who sows seeds of kindness enjoys a perpetual harvest.

- Kindness is the ability to love people more than they really deserve.

- A kindness done today is the surest way to a brighter tomorrow.

- The milk of human kindness never curdles.

- Kindness is the golden chain by which society is bound together.

- Kindness is a language which the deaf can hear and the blind can see.

- Kind words are like honey — sweet to the soul and healthy for the body.

- Your kindness will reward you, but your cruelty will destroy you.

- Learn to speak kind words — nobody resents them.

- Kindness pays most when you don't do it for pay.

- The kindness you spread today will be gathered up and returned to you tomorrow.

- A kindness put off until tomorrow may become only a bitter regret.

- How beautiful a day can be when kindness touches it.

- Kind words are short to speak, but their echoes are endless.

- Kind words do not wear out the tongue — so speak them.

- A kind word picks up a man when trouble weighs him down.

- There has never been an overproduction of kind words.

- The smallest act of kindness is worth more than the grandest intention. – *Oscar Wilde*

KNOWLEDGE

- Discussion is an exchange of knowledge; argument is an exchange of ignorance.

- Heads that are filled with knowledge and wisdom have little space left for conceit.

- Education should include knowledge of what to do with it.

- Education is not a head full of facts, but knowing *how* and *where* to find facts.

- What you don't know won't hurt you, but it may cause you to look pretty silly.

- Knowledge becomes wisdom only after it has been put to practical use.

- Knowledge, like lumber, is best when well-seasoned.

- Knowledge has to be improved, challenged, and increased constantly or it vanishes.

- No one is ever too old to learn, but many people keep putting it off anyway.

- Knowledge comes by taking things apart, but wisdom comes by putting things together.

- A smart person doesn't tell everything he knows, but he knows everything he tells.

- One part of knowledge consists in being ignorant of things that are not worth knowing.

- A little knowledge that acts is worth infinitely more than much knowledge that is idle.

- It's not so much what we know as how we use what we know.

- Knowledge is knowing a fact. Wisdom is knowing what to do with that fact.

- The only commodity on earth that does not deteriorate with use is knowledge.

- Knowledge is knowing a fact. Wisdom is knowing what to do with that fact.

- If you are unwilling to learn, no one can help you. If you are willing to learn, no one can stop you. – *ASU Psychology and Dept. of Education Bulletin*

- There are three kinds of people in the world: the uninformed, the misinformed and the well informed.

- The gateway to wisdom and knowledge are always open.

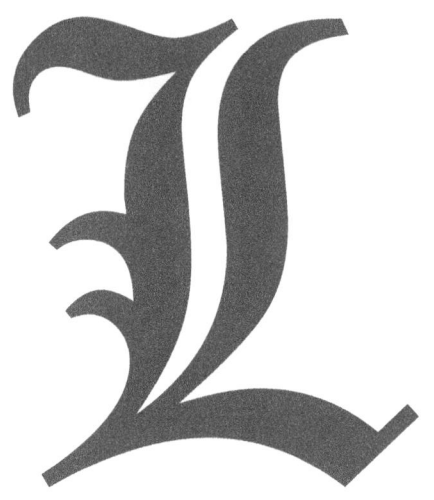

Lateness

- It is never too late to be what you might have become; it is never too late to mend.
- Every lateness gives us a staggering statistics in negative economic effect.
- Tardiness often robs us opportunity, and the dispatch of our forces.
- Those who start doing things late or at the eleventh hour are nimble in danger.

Laughter

- If you are too busy to laugh, you are too busy. – *Proverb*
- Laughter can conceal a heavy heart, but when the laughter ends, the grief remains.
- Laughter is the shock absorber that eases the blows of life.

- He who laughs last, laughs best.

LAZINESS

- Lazy people take food in their hand but don't even lift it to their mouth.

- Lazy people sleep soundly, but idleness leaves them hungry.

- Despite their desires, the lazy will come to ruin, for their hands refuse to work.

- Lazy people irritate their employers, like vinegar to the teeth or smoke in the eyes.

- Those too lazy to plow in the right season will have no food at the harvest.

- A lazy person is as bad as someone who destroys things.

- He who rests, rusts. – *German Proverb, "Wer rastet, der rostet"*

LEADERS

- The business of a leader is to turn weakness into strength, obstacles into stepping stones, and disaster into triumph.

- A good leader takes a little more than his share of the blame, a little less than his share of the credit.

- Followers do not usually go any farther than their leaders.

- A good leader inspires men to have confidence in him; a great leader inspires them to have confidence in themselves.

- Real leaders are ordinary people with extraordinary determination.

- Anyone who wants to be a leader must be the servant of those he wants to serve. – *Aminu Kano*

- Great leaders sometimes fail because of the failure to listen or question their mistake. – *Ameenah Gurib – Farik*

LEARNING

- Enough curiosity may enable you to learn, but too much of it can get you into trouble.

- A failure in life is one who lives and fails to learn.

- It is senseless to pay to educate a fool, since he has no heart for learning.

- Being ignorant is not so shameful as being unwilling to learn.

- What you don't know you can learn.

- Everyone I meet is in one way or the other my superior, in that I have something new to learn from him.

LIBERTY

- Liberty doesn't work as well in practice as it does in speeches.

- Every human being has the liberty to do that which is good, just, and honest.

- Liberty is the right to go just as far as the law allows.

- Personal liberty ends where public safety begins.

- Liberty is not a gift of God but a hard-won achievement with the help of God.

LIFE

- There are four steps to accomplishment: Plan purposefully. Prepare prayerfully. Proceed positively. Pursue persistently. – *William Arthur Ward*

- The future depends on what we do in the present. – *Mahatma Gandhi*

- It's the little moments that make life big.

- The greatest thing in the world is not so much where we are, but in what direction we are moving.

- All life is an experiment. The more experiments you make the better. – *Ralph Waldo Emerson*

- Celebrate your life no matter where it takes you — no matter how difficult — and know that it is only a transition. – *Kryon*

- No one finds life worth living; he must make it worth living!

- Life is 10 percent what you make it and 90 percent how you take it.

- If you break the rules in the game of life, the rules will eventually break you.

- A long life is a gift of God; a full and fruitful life is your own doing.

- The one thing certain about life is that we must leave it.

- Medical science is adding years to our lives, but it's up to us to add life to our years.

- Life is 10% of what happens to you and 90% of how you react to it. – *Charles Swindoll*

- Live in alignment with your values, vision, abilities and potential. – *Cherie Carter-Scott, Ph.D.*

- Your LIFE is a gift from GOD, what YOU do with it is your gift to GOD!!

- Look at the bright side of life.

- It is how I live my life that distinguishes me.

- While there's life, there's hope.

- I only have this one body so I will be kind to it and I will try to eat healthy food and exercise regularly.

- If you are unwilling to learn, no one can help you. If you are willing to learn, no one can stop you.

LISTENING

- You can win more friends with your ears than with your mouth.

- The Golden Rule of friendship is to listen to others as you would have them listen to you.

- Take a tip from nature — your ears aren't made to shut, but your mouth is!

- Always listen to the opinions of others. It may not do you much good but it will them.

- Opportunities are often missed because we are broadcasting when we should be listening.

- I have learned… that the head does not hear anything until the heart has listened, and that what the heart knows today the head will understand tomorrow.

LIVING

- When people speak evil of you, live so that no one will believe them.

- It's better to teach children the roots of labor than to hand them the fruits of yours.

- No one finds life worth living; he must make it worth living!

- You can live in this world but once, but if you live it right once is enough.

- An upright man can never be a downright failure.

- Man has learned to fly like a bird and swim like a fish — now all he needs to do is learn to live like a man.

- Wonderful things happen to us when we live expectantly, believe confidently, and pray affirmatively.

- It's better to live richly than to die rich.

- Riches won't help on the day of judgement, but right living can save you from death.

- One may go wrong in many directions but right in only one.

- The only way to be good is to obey God, love your fellowman, and hate the devil.

- Always do right; it will gratify some people and astonish others.

- Right living is better than high living — and cheaper.

- People who live right never get left.

- Go straight. Every crooked turn delays your arrival at success.

- The shortest route to success is the straight road.

- The straight and narrow path is the only one that has no traffic problems.

LONELINESS

- A bore keeps you from feeling lonely and makes you wish you were.

- ❦ Many people are lonely because they build walls and not bridges.

- ❦ Loneliness could be one of God's finest gifts. If a season of solitude is God's way to teach you to hear His song, don't you think it's worth it. – *Max Lucado*

- ❦ The reason many successful men are so lonely is because they sacrificed too many friends on the way up.

- ❦ The most lonely place in the world is the human heart when love is absent.

- ❦ To love others makes us happy; to love ourselves makes us lonely.

- ❦ Laugh and the world will laugh with you; think and you will almost die of loneliness.

- ❦ The surest way to be lonesome is to always tell the truth.

LOVE

- ❦ Love is the quest, marriage the conquest, divorce the inquest.

- You can give without loving, but you can't love without giving.

- Happiness is a healthy mental attitude, a grateful spirit, a clear conscience, and a heart full of love.

- Happiness is the conviction that we are loved in spite of ourselves.

- The loneliest place in the world is the human heart when love is absent.

- Love at first sight may be all right, but it might be wise to take a second look.

- Love is sharing a part of yourself with others.

- Love at first sight is often cured by a second look.

- He who falls in love with himself will have no rivals.

- Love is a fabric which never fades, no matter how often it is washed in the water of adversity and grief.

- Love intoxicates a man; marriage often sobers him.

- In your heart, my love has found a home and it will never die.

- Love is the beauty of the soul.

- Love is like the wind, you cannot see it; but you can feel it. –*Television*

- Love is the energy from which all people and things are made. You are connected to everything in your world through love. – *Brian L. Weiss, M.D.*

- Love others fully and with all your heart, do not fear, do not hold back. The more you give, the more will return to you. – *Brian L. Weiss, M.D.*

- Sacrifice is the biggest form of love. – *Mario Willis*

- To reach out with love, to do your best and not be so concerned with results or outcomes- that's the way to live. – *Brian L. Weiss, M.D.*

- If music is the food of love, play on. Give me enough of it. – *Shakespeare*

- We can love what we are, without hating what, and who, we are not. – *Kofi Annan*

LOYALTY

- A friend is always loyal, and a brother is born to help in time of need.

- Many will say they are loyal friends, but who can find one who is truly reliable?

- Never let loyalty and kindness leave you! Tie them around your neck as a reminder. Write them deep within your heart.

- Loyalty makes a person attractive. It is better to be poor than dishonest.

LUCK

- You can always tell luck from ability by its duration.

- Choice, not chance, determines destiny.

- Luck always seems to be against the man who depends on it.

- There may be luck in getting a job, but there's no luck involved in keeping it.

- Luck is good planning, carefully executed.

- Good luck is often with the man who doesn't include it in his plans.

- Industry is the mother of success — luck, a distant relative.

- Luck is what happens when preparation meets opportunity.

- The harder you work the luckier you get.

- Good luck happens when an opportunity presents itself. Meet it with preparedness. - *Deepak Chopra, M.D.*

LYING

- Telling lies about others is as harmful as hitting them with ax, wounding them with a sword, or shooting them with a sharp arrow.

- The crooked heart will not prosper; the lying tongue tumbles into trouble.

- The godly hate lies; the wicked cause shame and disgrace.

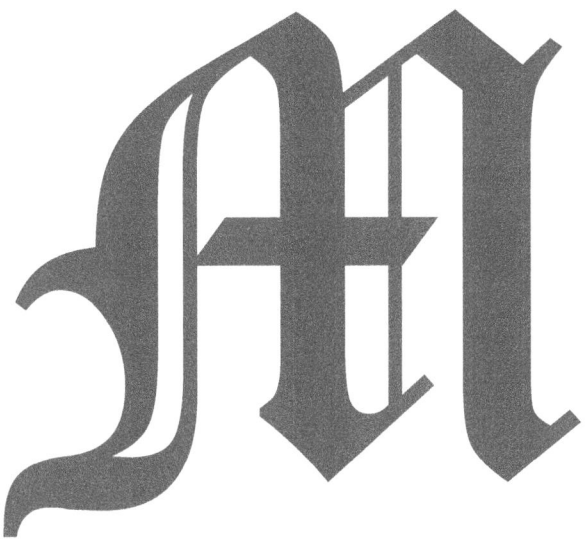

Marriage

- A marriage may be a holy wedlock or an unholy deadlock.

- A successful marriage requires falling in love many times, always with the same person. – *Mignon McLaughlin*

- Anybody who thinks marriage is a fifty-fifty proposition doesn't understand women or fractions.

- Marriage brings music into a man's life — he learns to play second fiddle.

- Marriage is a union of two hands, two hearts and two souls.

- Marriage is like arthritis. You have to learn to live with it.

- Marriage is too often a case where cupidity meets stupidity.

- Marriage may be inspired by music, soft words, and perfume; but its security is manifest in work, consideration, respect, and well-fried bacon.

- Marriage. It's a partnership between two people who decide to take the adventure of life together — sometimes crazy, sometimes routine, lots of times fun, but ALWAYS worth it.

- Marriages are made in heaven, but they are lived on earth.

- Nothing makes a marriage rust like distrust.

- One does not find happiness in marriage, but takes happiness into marriage.

- The argument you just won with your wife isn't over yet.

- The bonds of matrimony are like any other bond — they take a while to mature.

- The bonds of matrimony are worthless unless the interest is kept up.

- Too many people are finding it easier to get married than to stay married.

- What marriage needs is more open minds and fewer open mouths.

- Women need to receive caring, understanding and reassurance. Men need to receive trust.

Memory

- You always remember a kind deed — particularly if it was yours.

- Your creed may be interesting but your deeds are much more convincing.

- There are a lot of people who never forget a kind deed — if they did it!

- Education means developing the mind, not stuffing the memory.

- We commit the Golden Rule to memory and forget to commit it to life.

- It's strange how much better our memory becomes as soon as a friend borrows money from us.

- Creditors have a better memory than debtors.

- Every time you lend money to a friend you damage his memory.

- Anybody who tells you he never made a mistake in his life is probably relying on a poor memory — his or yours.

- Three things indicate we are getting old. First, the loss of memory — and we can't remember the other two.

- To err is human, to forgive, divine. – *Alexander Pope*

MIND

- Quite often when a man thinks his mind is getting broader, it is only his conscience stretching.

- Conversation is an exercise of the mind, but gossiping is merely an exercise of the tongue.

- Crime begins in the mind. A man has to think wrong before he acts wrong.

- Hatred is cancer of the intellect.

- Hate pollutes the mind.

- Your brain becomes a mind when it's fortified with knowledge.

- A mature mind is not always found in a mature body.

- If a cluttered desk is a sign of a cluttered mind, just what does an empty desk mean?

- At a certain age some people's minds close up — they live on their intellectual fat.

- Only hungry minds can become educated.

- A human mind is a terrible thing to waste.

- Great minds discuss ideas, average minds discuss events, small minds discuss people.

- Great minds have purposes; others have wishes.

- Small minds are the first to condemn great ideas.

- The mind is like the stomach. It's not how much you put into it that counts, but how much it digests.

- Your mind is a sacred enclosure into which nothing harmful can enter except by your permission.

- An open mind is sometimes too porous to hold a conviction.

- Like swift water an active mind never stagnates.

- The mind, like a parachute, functions only when open.

- Think high and you will grow. Think low and you will fall below. Think that you can and you will. It is all in the state of mind.

MISTAKES

- The quickest way to get a lot of individual attention is to make a big mistake.

- The fellow who is always jumping to conclusions isn't always sure of a happy landing.

- The least expensive education is to profit from the mistakes of others — and ourselves.

- An error doesn't become a mistake until you refuse to correct it.

- Those who fear the future are likely to fumble the present.

- Freedom is not worth having if it does not include the freedom to make mistakes.

- Getting married is one mistake every man should make.

- The man who never makes a mistake must get awfully tired doing nothing.

- He who makes the same mistake over and over again learns to do at least one thing well.

- Anyone who corrects all his mistakes is probably writing his memoirs.

- The greatest mistake you can make in life is to be continually fearing you will make one. – *Elbert Hubbard*

- Few things in life are more difficult for some of us than admitting a mistake.

- It is easier to hide mistakes than to prevent their consequences.

- Most people make the mistake of looking too far ahead for things close by.

- A man must be big enough to admit his mistakes, smart enough to profit from them, and strong enough to correct them. – *John C. Maxwell*

- It is the highest form of self-respect to admit mistakes and make amends for them.

- Silence never makes any blunders.

- The three most difficult words to speak are, *"I was mistaken."*

- Make the mistakes of yesterday your lessons for today.

- Be willing to admit that you're wrong or have made a mistake. It's the only way to learn. – *Christiane Northrup, M.D.*

MODESTY

- The more a man knows, the more modest he is inclined to be.

- The greater the man's talent, the more becoming his modesty.

- Modesty is the art of enhancing your charm by pretending not to be aware of it.

- A person shouldn't be too modest. A light hidden under a bushel is seldom seen and less often appreciated.

- Modesty is the triumph of mind over flatter.

- A modest man is generally admired, if people ever hear of him.

- The more a man knows, the more he is inclined to be modest.

Money

- Money is energy in an exchange of services. How much do you depend on what you believe you deserve. – *Louise L. Hay*

- Money is only money, not a substitute for happiness.

- The greatest secret to making money and being successful is helping other people making money and be successful. – *Deepak Chopra. M.D*

- The earnings of the godly enhance their lives, but evil people squander their money on sin.

- Trust in your money and down you go! But the godly flourish like leaves in spring.

- How much money is enough? Foe each and every one of us, that amount is different, unique as a fingerprint. Seek and celebrate all that you can create, than you're meant to have. That will be enough. – *Suzie Orman*

- If you want money in your life, then you must welcome it, be open to it, and treat it with respect. Your beliefs and your attitudes are what make you feel rich and free to trust yourself knowing that you will always take the right actions with your money. – *Suze Orman*

- Money in its own has only the power to languish. You are the one who gives it the power to grow. Remember, your money is only as powerful… as you are powerful over your money. – *Suze Orman*

- What happens to your money directly affects the quality of your life, not your stockbroker's life, but your life. – *Suze Orman*

- Money is the root of all evils.

- Money maketh a man.

Mothers

- Through a mother's loving eyes, her children see the world. Through a mother's gentle words, they learn both trust and sharing.

- The hand that rocks the cradle rules the world.

- Mother's love is the fuel that enables a normal human being to do the impossible.

- Mother is the heartbeat in the home; and without her, there seems to be no heart throb.

Mutualism

- An iron sharpens iron, so a friend sharpens a friend.

- It is a privilege to share my thoughts with others and for them to share their thoughts with me.

- Left hand washes the right hand while the right hand washes the left hand and they both become clean.

❦ If someone avoids you, let them be undisturbed. One day they will understand that your symbiotic relationship is mutualism, not parasitism.

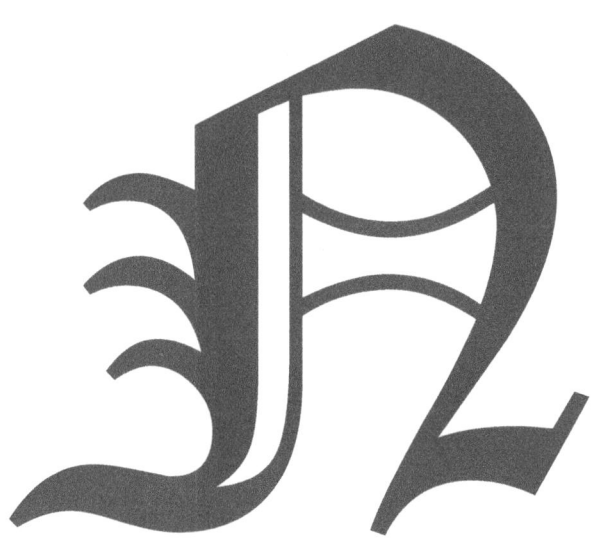

NATURE

- An echo is nature's instant replay.

- By nature, all men are much alike, but by education they become different.

- Nature couldn't make us perfect, so she did the next best thing: she made us blind to our faults.

- Nature makes blunders too — she often gives the biggest mouths to those who have the least to say.

NEEDS

- The world's greatest need is an assurance of tomorrow.

- Man's greatest need is something to feel important about.

- Above all, we need tranquility without tranquilizers.

- What this world needs are fewer rules and more good examples.

※ What the world needs is peace that passes all misunderstanding.

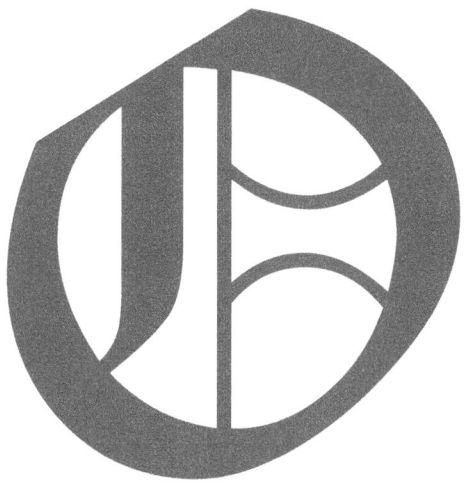

OBESITY

- Like charity, obesity begins at home.

- He who indulges bulges.

- Obesity is surplus gone to waist.

- Every cure of obesity must begin with these three essential precepts: discretion in eating, moderation in sleeping, and exercise.

OBSTACLE

- Scale the wall of negativity and self-doubt and refuse to allow any obstacle to separate you from the attainment of your dreams. – *Keith D. Harrell*

- When an obstacle arises in one of your relationships, know that you can replace any fearful feelings with those of love. – *Deepak Chopra, M.D.*

- Remove the obstacles. Untangle the clutter that's standing between you and the productive, fulfilling life. – *Julie Morgenstern*

- One's life shrinks or expands in proportion to one's courage. Success is often the result of taking a misstep in the right direction. Only when you are no longer afraid do you begin to live.

- Obstacles are what you see when you take your eyes off your goals.

Offerings

- Each man should give what he had decided in his heart to give, not reluctantly or under compulsion for God loves a cheerful giver. – *2 Corinthians 9:7*

- As the purse is emptied the heart is filled. – *Victor Hugo*

- No man is above the law and no man is below it; nor do we ask any man's permission when we require him to obey it. – *Theodore Roosevelt*

- Morality cannot be legislated, but behavior can be regulated. Judicial decrees may not change the heart, but they can restrain the heartless. – *Martin Luther King, Jr.*

OPINIONS

- Most people, when they come to you for advice, want their opinions strengthened, not corrected.

- People generally have too many opinions and not enough convictions.

- Every man has a right to his opinion, but no man has a right to be wrong about the facts.

- Facts do not change; feelings do.

- Public opinion is what folks think.

- It's a lot easier to form an opinion when you have only a few of the facts.

- The man who has strong opinions and always says what he thinks is courageous — and friendless.

- A wise man gives other people's opinions as much weight as he does his own.

- A great deal of laziness of mind is called liberty of opinion.

- The man who has a good opinion of himself is usually a poor judge.

- One of the most difficult secrets for a man to keep is his opinion of himself.

- Be confident enough to be able to voice your opinions without fear of recrimination. As such, you will inspire the same action in others. – *Deepak Chopra, M.D.*

- We need to appreciate that we can have different shades of opinion. – *Uhuru Kenyatta*

Opportunity

- There is far more opportunity than there is ability.

- Good behavior gets a lot of credit that really belongs to a lack of opportunity.

- When opportunity knocks a grumbler complains about the noise.

- Sometimes it's difficult to know who's knocking — opportunity or temptation.

- There are opportunities even in the most difficult moments. – *Wangari Maathal*

- In the middle of difficulty lies opportunity. – *Albert Einstein*

- Opportunity usually knocks but once, and that may be the reason it has a better reputation than other knockers.

- A wise man will make more opportunities than he finds.

- We are continually faced by great opportunities brilliantly disguised as insolvable problem.

- When you have a chance to embrace an opportunity, give it a big hug.

- The reason a lot of people can't find opportunity is that it is often disguised as hard work.

- Great opportunities come to those who make the most of small ones.

- The gates of opportunity swing on four hinges: initiative, insight, industry, and integrity.

- Those who wait for opportunities to turn up usually find themselves turned down.

- Never waste time reflecting on opportunities you have missed. While thus reflecting you might miss some more.

- Between tomorrow's dream and yesterday's regret is today's opportunity.

- Once an opportunity has passed, it cannot be caught.

- We are seldom able to see an opportunity until it has ceased to be one.

- For some reason a pessimist always complains about the noise when opportunity knocks.

- The reason some men don't go very far in life is that they sidestep opportunity and shake hands with temptation.

Optimists

- Better a bald head than none at all.

- You can't have rosy thoughts about the future when your mind is full of the blues about the past.

- We all hope for the best, but an optimist actually expects to get it.

- Optimism is man's passport to a better tomorrow.

- If you see good in everything, you may be an optimist. On the other hand, you may be nuts.

- Have you noticed that an optimist is always able to see the bright side of other people's troubles?

- The greatest of all optimists is the man who proclaims we live in the best of worlds. The pessimist fears that such is true.

- The optimist says his glass is half full; the pessimist says his glass is half empty.

- An optimist tells you to cheer up, especially when things are going his way.

- An optimist is often as wrong as the pessimist, but he has a lot more fun.

- Optimism is often the determination to see more in something than is there.

- Optimists count their blessings; pessimists discount theirs.

- To the optimist, a fireplace is a center of warmth and beauty. To the pessimist, it is a source of smoke and ashes.

- I do not know how long I have on this earth, but I will try hard to make the most of each and every day.

- I see the glass as half-full.

- Hope for the best while prepared for the worst.

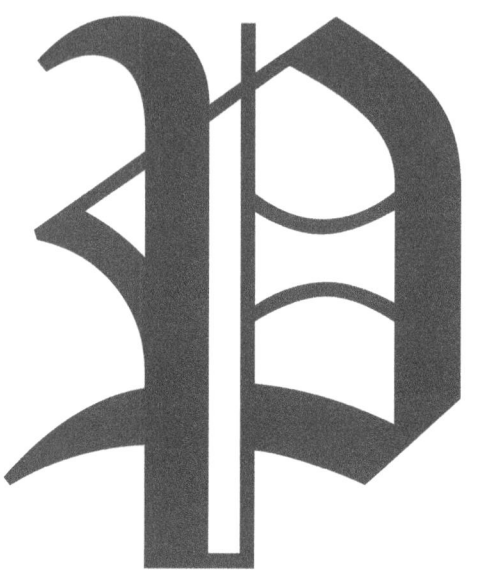

Parenthood

- Train up a child in the way he should go: and when he is old, he will not depart from it.

- The greatest thing a father can do for his children is to love their mother. – *Jos Mcdowell*

- If you want your children to keep their feet on the ground, put some responsibility on their shoulders. – *Abigail Van Buren*

- With your own kids, you have the chance to rewrite history to parent them as you wish you had been parented. Thus does your own re-parenting occur. You release the future as your release the past. – *Marianne Williamson*

Partnership

- Understand the power of partnership, whenever you work with one or more synergistically, your power becomes exponentially greater than it could ever be individually. – *Christiane Northrup, M.D.*

- A true partnership provides a safe place to take risks, it also encourages mutual growth and evolution. – *Christiane Northrup, M.D.*

- Part of working on yourself is learning how to support another person in being the best they can be. Partners are meant to help each other access the highest parts within themselves. – *Marianne Williamson*

Patience

- You cannot run faster than your legs can carry you.

- Better be patient on the road than a patient in the hospital.

- Patience, forbearance, and understanding are companions to contentment.

- Be patient with the faults of others; they may have to be patient with yours.

- Happy homes are built with blocks of patience.

- The true measure of a man is the height of his ideals, the breadth of his sympathy, the depth of his convictions, and the length of his patience.

- The trouble with people today is that they want to get to the promised land without going through the wilderness.

- Patience is a quality that is most needed when it is exhausted.

- Patience is the art of concealing your impatience.

- You should bear with people because they have to bear with you.

- Patience is often bitter, but its fruit is sweet.

- Nothing worthwhile ever happens in a hurry — so be patient!

- Nothing worthwhile is achieved without patience, labor, and disappointment.

- Patience is the greatest of all shock absorbers. About the only thing you can get in a hurry is trouble.

- True patience means waiting without worrying.

- Patience is the companion of wisdom. – *Saint Augustine*

- Good things come to those who wait.

- Patience truly is a virtue, and it is one attribute that we all have to perfect in one form or another. Instead of getting impatient, try doing a short meditation— breathe deeply and think pleasant thoughts. – *Sylvia Browne*

Patriotism

- True patriotism is your conviction that this country is superior to all others because you were born in it!

- A patriot is the fellow who is always ready and willing to lay down your life for his country.

- A patriot is a man working for his country's future instead of boasting its past.

- Patriotism is your conviction that this country is superior to all other countries because you were born in it. – *George Bernard Shaw*

PEACE

- Peace may cost as much as war, but it's a better buy.

- When a man finds no peace within himself, it is useless to seek it elsewhere.

- Peace is not made in documents, but in the hearts of men.

- Peace won by the compromise of principles is a short-lived achievement.

- What the nations of the world need is a peace conference with the "Prince of Peace."

- Peace can be achieved by the substitution of reason for force, right for might, law for war.

- The key to lasting peace is to rely less on arms and more on heads.

- Avoid the enticement to mean or argue. Allow others to be right period. As for as your concerned, be peaceful with everyone you encounter. – *Tavis Smiley*

- Peace is much more than the absence of war and violence; it is a condition onto itself the goal at this point must be the creation of peace. Without love, there is no peace. Where love is absent, war of some kind is inevitable. – *Marianne Williamson*

❧ Better a dry crust eaten in peace than a house filled with feasting and conflict.

❧ Everything you are against can be restated in a way that puts toy in support. Instead of being at war, be at peace; instead of being against poverty, be for prosperity. – *Dr. Wayne W. Dyer*

❧ Avoid the enticement to mean or argue. Allow others to be right period. As far as you're concerned, be peaceful with everyone you encounter. – *Tavis Smiley*

Persistence

❧ He is like a rock in the sea, unshaken, stands his ground.

❧ The mere absence of war is not peace. – *John F. Kennedy*

❧ Where there is peace, God is. – *George Herbert*

- All great achievements require time. – *Maya Angelou*

- Pick up a snake. You are going to get bit.

- The greatest accomplishment is not in never falling but in rising again after you fall. – *Vince Lombardi*

- Old soldiers never die, they just fade away.

- Hope is the dream of a waking man.

Perfection

- You will never have a friend if you must have one without a fault.

- None of us is perfect, but the worst of it is that many of us are impossible.

- The only way a man can attain perfection is to follow the advice he gives to others.

- A man who knows his imperfections is just about as perfect as anyone can be.

- We all know it isn't human to be perfect, and too many of us take advantage of it.

- The person who tells you how perfect he thinks you are will lie to others too.

PERSEVERANCE

- There are four steps to accomplishment: Plan purposefully. Prepare prayerfully. Proceed positively. Pursue persistently. – *William Arthur Ward*

- The thing to try when all else fails is again.

- The man who gets ahead is the man who does more than is necessary — and keeps on doing it.

- If you have tried your hand at something and failed, the next best thing is to try your head.

- Falling down doesn't make you a failure, but staying down does.

- Failure is the path of least persistence.

- Faith either moves mountains or tunnels through.

- The secret of happiness is to learn to accept the impossible, to do without the indispensable, and to bear the intolerable.

- The trouble with some people is that during trying times they stop trying.

- Perseverance has been defined as sticking to something you're not stuck on.

- Perseverance is the result of a strong will. Obstinacy is the result of a strong "won't."

- Some men may succeed because they are destined to, but most men succeed because they are determined to.

- The basic rules for success may be defined as follows: Know what you want. Find out what it takes to get it. Act on it and persevere.

- If at first you don't succeed, try, try again. Then quit. There's no point in making a fool of yourself.

- To succeed — do the best you can, where you are, with what you have.

Pessimists

- The greatest of all optimists is the man who proclaims we live in the best of worlds. The pessimist fears that such is true.

- Optimists count their blessings; pessimists discount theirs.

- Many people aren't pessimists — they're merely discontented optimists.

- One reason a pessimist isn't very well-liked is that he so often has the opportunity to say, *"I told you so."*

- A pessimist burns his bridges before he gets to them.

- With a choice of two evils, the pessimist takes both. – *Oscar Wilde*

- The pessimist is a person who absorbs sunshine and radiates gloom.

- A pessimist actually thinks the chief purpose of sunshine is to cast shadows.

- Nothing worries the pessimist like the optimist who says there's nothing to worry about.

- To the pessimistic patient, "consultation" means that his doctor has decided to call in an accomplice.

- It is impossible to be prayerful and pessimistic at the same time.

- A successful man is one who has the horsepower of an optimist and the emergency brakes of a pessimist.

PLAN

- Those who fail to plan, plan to fail.

- Plans succeed through good counsel; don't go to war without good advice. – *Proverbs 20:18*

- Good planning and hard work lead to prosperity, but hasty shortcuts lead to poverty. – *Proverbs 21:5*

- A goal without a plan is just a wish.

- An hour of planning can save you 10 hours of doing. – *Dale Carnegie*

- If the plan doesn't work change the plan, not the goal.

PLEASURE

- The trouble with mixing business and pleasure is that pleasure usually comes out on top.

- Two vastly underrated pleasures are scratching and sneezing.

- The greatest pleasure in life is doing what other people say can't be done.

- The greatest and noblest pleasure men can have in this world is to discover new truths, and the next is to shake off old prejudices. – *Frederick the Great*

- A toast: MAY ALL YOUR PLEASURES BECOME HABITS.

- Work is the meat of life; pleasure, the dessert. – *B. C. Forbes*

- There are two things that give pleasure; sex and scientific work. But, the second lasts much.

- Do something just for fun. Pleasure is one of life's essential nutrients. – *Cheryl Richardson*

- Resolve to perform what you ought; perform without fail what you resolve. – *Benjamin Franklin*

POLITICS

- A good place to keep your friends is out of politics.

- Politics is the science of who gets what, when, and why!

- Political speeches are usually just baloney disguised as food for thought.

- Political differences are wholesome. It's political indifference that hurts.

- It takes two things to conduct a successful political campaign: hot issues and cold cash.

- The most important thing in politics is sincerity, whether you mean it or not.

- The guy who never votes is the first to tell you what's wrong with the government.

- The whole purpose of any political campaign is to stay calm, cool, and elected.

- Nothing is politically right when it is morally wrong.

- The toughest part of politics is to satisfy the voter without giving him what he wants.

- Politics is the only profession in which a man can make a living solely by bragging.

- A good political candidate needs three things — the patient understanding of a bartender, the political knowledge of a barber, and the assurance of a cab driver.

- Before you undertake to change a man's religion or politics, be sure you've got something better to offer him.

- A political war is one in which everybody shoots from the lip.

POPULARITY

- Popularity is a do-it-yourself job.

- Your popularity will depend on *how* you treat your friends — and how often!

- Popularity is a form of success that's seldom worth the things we have to do in order to attain it.

- Popularity is a matter of whether people like you wherever you go or like it whenever you leave.

- To be extremely popular, one must be more tactful than truthful.

- When a person sells principles for popularity, he is soon bankrupt.

- Tact will make you popular, provided you endure being taught many things you already know.

POVERTY

- The two great tests of character are wealth and poverty. – *Charles A. Beard*

- Friends are like a priceless treasure; he who has none is a social pauper.

- The chief reward for idleness is poverty.

- A man is truly poor, not when he *has* nothing, but when he *does* nothing.

- Poverty is no disgrace, but ignorance is.

- Being poor is no sin, but what good is it?

- Poverty is no disgrace — provided no one knows it.

- It's no shame to be poor, and, besides, the salesmen leave you alone.

- Poverty isn't dishonorable in itself — but it is dishonorable when it comes from idleness, intemperance, extravagance, and folly. – *Plutarch*

- Poverty is no disgrace, but that's about all you can say in its favor.

- Mandatory retirement is another form of compulsory poverty.

POWER

- Men of genius are admired; men of wealth are envied; men of power are feared; but only men of character are trusted. – *Alfred Adler*

- Knowledge is power only when it is turned on.

- Power will either burn a man out or light him up.

- The greatest power for good is the power of example.

- There is more power in the open hand than in the clenched fist. – *Herbert Newton*

- A man with compassion wields more power than a man with muscle.

- Prayer provides power, poise, peace, and purpose.

- No one can give you power. It is yours to take! – *MKO Abiola*

- Perceive things as equitable, then anticipate justice prevailing. – *Cherie Carter-Scott, Ph.D.*

- Smile and laugh often! Each day, find something happy, joyful, and funny about life- smile and laugh, smile and laugh, and smile and laugh again. – *Keith D. Harrell*

- Words make a powerful impact and they're not easily forgotten. Wounds inflicted by words of anger or hate can last a very long time. – *Brian L. Weiss, M.D.*

- The people in power are no match for the power of the people.

- When you recognize and acknowledge your personal power, you no longer need to feel superior or inferior to anyone else. – *Deepak Chopra, M.D.*

- Jealousy and competitiveness are emotions that in a small amount are normal but in big doses are the signs of an unhappy, bitter person.

Praise

- It's easy to keep from being a bore. Just praise the person to whom you're talking.

- If you're not mature enough to take criticism; you're too immature for praise.

- Insincere praise is worse than no praise at all.

- It is not he who searches for praise who finds it.

- The man who sings his own praises may have the right tune but the wrong words.

- It is usually best to be generous with praise, but cautious with criticism.

- Be the first to praise and the first to deserve praise.

- Praise does wonders for a person's hearing.

- When good becomes better, the best is our goal.

Prayer

- Do not pray for easy lives; pray to be stronger men! Do not pray for tasks equal to your power, pray for powers equal to your tasks… – *Phillip Brooks*

- If you don't have faith, pray anyway. If you don't understand or believe the words you're saying, pray anyway. Prayer can start faith, particularly if you pray aloud. And even the most imperfect prayer is an attempt to reach God. – *Gary Grant*

- Any concern too small to be made into a prayer is too small to be made into a burden. – *Corrie ten Boom*

- In prayer it is better to have a heart without words than words without a heart. – *John Bunyan*

- Lord, when we are wrong, make us willing to change and when we are right make us easy to live with. – *Peter Marhshall*

- More things are wrought by prayer than this world dreams of. – *Alfred Lord Tennyson*

- Prayer is not overcoming God's reluctance; it is laying hold of his highest willingness. – *RC Trench*

- I have found the perfect antidote for fear. Whenever it sticks up its ugly face I clobber it with prayer… – *Dale Evans Rogers*

Prejudice

- What some people call a conviction may be just a prejudice.

- An opinion is usually a prejudice with a few unrelated facts.

- There is nothing so easy to acquire and so difficult to drop as prejudice.

- Prejudice is a lazy man's substitute for thinking.

- No prejudice has ever been able to prove its case in the court of reason.

- A prejudiced person is someone who's too stubborn to admit you're right!

- Prejudice is when you deicide a fellow is a stinker before you even meet him.

- Prejudice cannot see things that are, because it is always looking for things that aren't.

PREVENTION

- An ounce of prevention is worth than a pound of cure. – *Benjamin Franklin*

- Care is an absolute. Prevention is the ideal.

- True prevention is not waiting for bad things to happen, it is preventing things from happening in the first place.

Pride

- Unfriendly people care only about themselves; they lash out at common sense.

- Pride leads to conflict; those who take advise are wise.

- Haughtiness goes before destruction; humility precedes honor. – *Proverbs 18:12*

- Pride goes before destruction and haughtiness before a fall.

- A fool's proud talk becomes a rod that beats him, but the words of the wise keep them safe. – *Proverbs 14:3*

- Pride goes before a fall.

Principles

- Compromise is always wrong when it means sacrificing a principle.

- A man without principle never draws much interest.

- No man is better than his principles.

- It's easier to fight for principles than to live up to them. – *Alfred Adler*

- It takes a wise man to know when he is fighting for a principle, or merely defending a prejudice.

Procrastination

- Procrastination is a lazy man's apology. – *Chinua Achebe*

- The best time to do something worthwhile is between yesterday and tomorrow.

- One can conquer a bad habit easier today than tomorrow.

- The kindness we resolve to show tomorrow cures no headaches today.

- No one is ever too old to learn, but many people keep putting it off anyway.

- The lazier a man is, the more he Is going to do tomorrow.

- Procrastination is the thief of time. So are a lot of other big words.

- Never put off until tomorrow what you can order someone else to do today.

- Some tasks have to be put off dozens of times before they completely slip your mind.

- Procrastination is the fertilizer that makes difficulties grow.

- What you put off today, you'll probably put off tomorrow too.

- Sometimes it is better to put off until tomorrow what you are likely to mess up today.

- The main thing that comes to a man who waits is regret for having waited.

- Procrastination is the grave in which opportunity is buried. – *Alyce Cornyn-Selby*

- A lot of folks postpone until tomorrow those things they should have done several days ago.

- A procrastinator is one who puts off until tomorrow the things he has already put off until today.

- About the only thing that comes to him who waits is old age.

- No one can build a reputation on what he's going to do tomorrow.

- Hard work is usually an accumulation of easy things that should have been done last week.

- Whatever you have to do, do it quickly, defer not till tomorrow what the morning can accomplish.

Proficiency

- You stop being good when you stop being better.

- Mastering others is strength. Mastering oneself makes you fearless. – *Lao Tzu*

- When you serve your passions, proficiency gradually takes over and becomes habitual.

PROGRESS

- A conceited person never gets anywhere because he thinks he is already there.

- It is not enough to make progress; we must make it in the right direction.

- The price of progress is change, and it is taking just about all we have.

- Progress is going around in the same circle — but faster.

- It's our desire to get ahead of each other that creates progress — and friction!

- Progress is largely a matter of discarding old worries and taking on new ones.

- Progress has little to do with speed, but much to do with direction. – *Timber Hawkeye*

- True progress consists not so much in increasing our needs as in diminishing our wants.

- Coming together is a beginning, keeping together is progress, working together is success. – *Henry Ford*

- Bloom where you are planted. – *Mother Jones*

- Forward ever, backward never. – *Mbadikwe*

- Smiles reach hard to reach places.

- He who stops being better, stops being good.

- Progress always involves risk, but you can't steal second base and keep your foot off first. – *Frederick B. Wilcox*

- Remember that there is no stagnation in life, you are either moving up or sliding down.

- To keep progressing, you must learn, commit, and do — learn, commit, and do — and learn, commit, and do all over again. – *Stephen R. Covey*

- When good becomes better, the best is our goal.

Promises

- Promises may get friends, but it is performance that keeps them.

- Promises are like money — easier made than kept.

- Some people stand on the promises; others just sit on the premises.

- Promises are only as dependable as the individuals who make them.

- One thing you can give and still keep is your word.

- I had rather do and not promise, than promise and not do. – *Arthur Warwick*

Prosperity

- We learn some things from prosperity, but we learn many more from adversity.

- Education is an ornament in prosperity and a refuge in adversity. – *Aristotle*

- Prosperity makes friends; adversity tries them.

- People become well-to-do by doing what they do well.

- Sometimes virtue and prosperity have trouble living together.

- A no time is self-control more difficult than in time of success.

- If you put something in its proper home, you'll feel so good when you go to look for it — and there it is.
  – *Julie Morgenstern*

Protection

- El Eyon, most strong and highest God, may it please thee to change the heart of my enemies and opposers that they may do me good instead of evil as thou didist in the days of Abraham when he Called upon thee by this holy name, Amen Selah.

- I am made in the image and likeness of Christ Nothing harmful shall happen to me. I am protected.

- Protect me according to thy good will and pleasure from violent sudden and unnatural death and from all other evil accidents and severe bodily affections. For thou art my help and my God and thine is the power and glory, Amen Selah.

- Starting a quarrel is like opening a floodgate, so stop before a dispute breaks out.

Prudence

- A prudent person foresees danger and takes precautions.

- Prudence is the footprint of wisdom.

- In matters of conscience, first thoughts are best. In matters of prudence, last thoughts are the best.

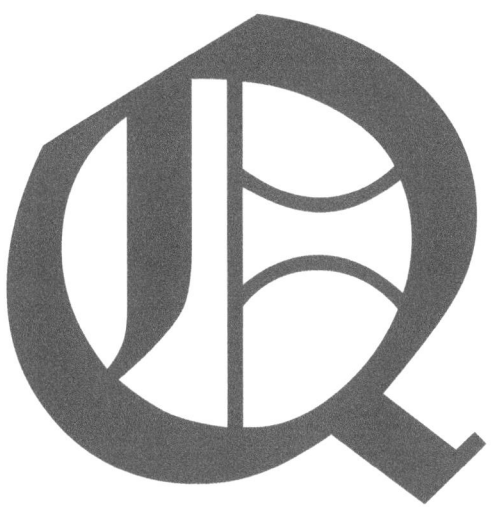

QUESTIONING

- I see things and I say "Why?" But I dream things that never were and I say "Why not?" – *George Bernard Shaw*

- It is better to debate a question without settling it than to settle a question without debating it. – *Joseph Joubert*

- Hypothetical questions get hypothetical answers. – *Joan Base*

- Question authority, but raise your hand first. – *Bob Thaves*

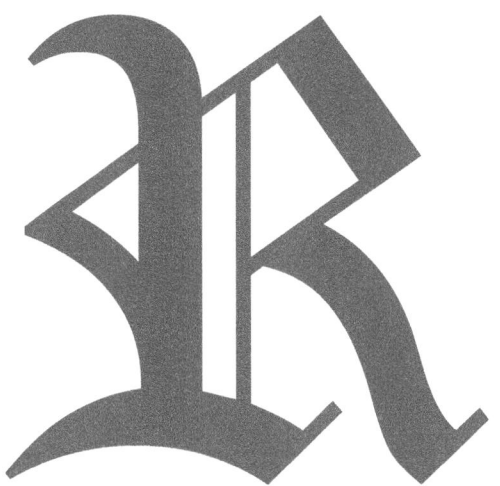

Relationship

- Celebrate every relationship you've ever had. For better or worse, your relationships are your best teachers. – *Christiane Northrup. M.D.*

- By focusing on relationships and results rather than time and methods, you can become a listener, a trainer, and a consultant to those in your sphere of influence. Your effectiveness- and that of those around you- will increase dramatically. – *Stephen R. Covey*

- In this world, you learn through relationships, not things. You can't take your things with you when you leave. – *Brian L. Weiss, M.D.*

- And one standing alone can be attacked and defeated, but two can stand back-to-back and conquer; three is even better, for a triple-braided cord is not easily broken.

- It is better to be alone, than in bad company.

- Education will broaden a narrow mind, but there is no known cure for a big head.

- It isn't easy for an idea to squeeze itself into a head that is filled with prejudice.

- Nothing dies quicker than a new idea in a closed mind.

- The most difficult thing to open is a closed mind.

- A narrow mind and an open mouth usually go together.

- A lot of trouble is caused by combining a narrow mind with a wide mouth.

RELIABILITY

- A person who promises a gift but doesn't give it is like clouds and wind that bring no rain.

- An unreliable messenger stumbles into trouble, but a reliable messenger brings healing.

- The shifts of fortune test the reliability of friends.

- Reliability is the quality that leads others not just to believe you but to believe in you.

Repentance

- It takes more courage to repent than to keep on sinning.

- To grieve over sin is one thing; to repent is another.

- It seems that more people repent of their sins from fear of punishment than from a change of heart.

- To do it no more is the truest repentance. – *Martin Luther*

Reputation

- Reputation is precious, but character is priceless.

- Reputation is what you need to get a job; character is what you need to keep it.

- A good past is the best thing a man can use for a future reference.

- Take care of your character and your reputation will take care of itself.

- Everyone should fear death until he has something that will live on after his death.

- White lies are likely to leave black marks on a man's reputation.

- A man has three names: the name he inherits, the name his parents gave him, and the name he makes for himself.

- The best inheritance parents can leave a child is a good name.

- No one can build a reputation on what he's going to do tomorrow.

- No human being is rich enough to buy back his past.

- The easiest thing to get, but the most difficult thing to get rid of, is a bad reputation.

- It is generally agreed that a man is known by the company he keeps out of!

- Your reputation can be damaged by the opinions of others. Only you yourself can damage your character.

- Many men would turn over a new leaf if they could tear out some of the old pages.

- People may try to ruin your reputation, and this can hurt. But remember, it can only hurt your feelings. The world will forget, so don't how on to bad publicity or what others say. You and God know the truth, so let the rest of it go. – *Sylvia Browne*

Resentment

- A stone is heavy and sand is weighty, but the resentment caused by a fool is even heavier.

- Resentment is like drinking poison and then hoping it will kill your enemies.

- Anger, resentment and jealousy don't change the heart of others, it only changes yours.

Respect

- Demanding respect is like chasing a butterfly. Chase it, and you'll never catch it. Sit still, and it may light on your shoulder. – *Max Lucado*

- A person with good sense is respected; a treacherous person is headed for destruction.

- Be respectful.

- Treat your body with respect by feeding it nourishing and nutritious foods. If you're good to your body, it will be good to you. – *Sylvia Browne*

- Respect yourself. You're the best judge of what's right. – *Cheryl Richardson*

Responsibility

- Our actions are our own; their consequences are not.

- Freedom is a package deal — with it comes responsibilities and consequences.

- Responsibility develops some men and ruins others.

- Those who shrink from responsibilities keep on shrinking in other ways too.

- Some people recognize their responsibilities in time to dodge them.

- You cannot escape the responsibilities of tomorrow by evading them today.

- A man's work is a portrait of himself.

- Learning to delegate responsibility to other skilled and trained people enables you to devote your energy to other high-leverage activities. Delegation means growth, both for individuals and organizations. – *Stephen R. Covey*

- Be responsible.

- You may not have been responsible for your heritage, but you are responsible for your future.

REVENGE

- Revenge may be sweet, but not when you are on the receiving end.

- The longest odds in the world are those against getting even with someone.

- You will never get ahead of anyone as long as you're trying to get even with him.

- The world has always acted on the principle that one good kick deserves another.

Riches

- Be kind to people until you make your first million. After that, people will be kind to you.
- No man is rich enough to buy back his past.
- No amount of riches can atone for poverty of character.
- Riches are a golden key that opens every door, save that of heaven.
- In your search for riches, don't lose the things that money can't buy.
- It is what we value, not what we have, that makes us rich.

Righteousness

- Garments of righteousness never go out of style.

- Some people are always greedy for more, but the godly love to give!

- Where there is no thirst for righteousness, the sermon is always "dry."

- Whoever pursues righteousness and unfailing love will find life, righteousness, and honor.

- The righteous despise the unjust; the wicked despise the godly.

- The time is always right to do what is right. – *Martin Luther King, Jr.*

- Do the right thing…especially when no one is watching. – *Cherie Carter-Scott, Ph.D.*

- It is better to light one candle than to cause the darkness. – *Confucius*

- Keep your face to the sunshine and you cannot see a shadow. – *Hellen Keller*

RISK

- Take a risk. You have the power within to move the mountains. – *Cheryl Richardson*

- What's the big hurry? You're not ever going to get it done, so what are you racing toward?

- Every single activity that you're involved in is for one purpose only, and that is to give you a moment of joy. Lighten up. Laugh more. Appreciate more. All is well. – *Abraham-Hicks*

- Greedy people try to get rich quick but don't realize they're headed for poverty.

RUMORS

- It's easier to float a rumor than to sink one.

- We still can't understand how rumors without a leg to stand on gets around so fast.

- A rumor is like a check — never endorse it till you're sure it's genuine.

- All rumors should be fitted with girdles to keep them from spreading.

- A groundless rumor often covers a lot of ground.

- The slanderer differs from the assassin only in that he murders the reputation instead of the body.

- Everybody likes to hear the truth — especially about somebody else.

- Rumors will always abound, and the more you do in life, the more you will be a target. If you're doing what you feel God wants, the rumors won't hurt you but also be careful that you are not the one starting or spreading rumors. – *Sylvia Browne*

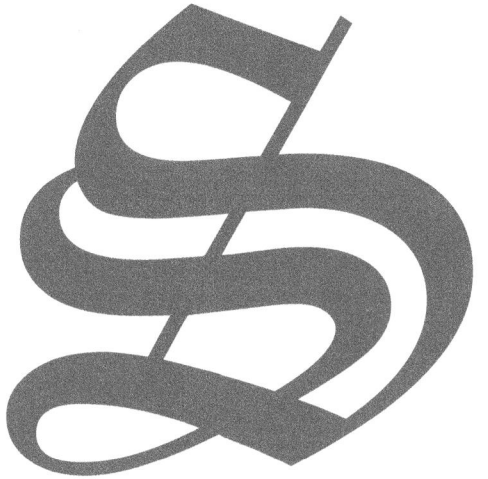

Sacrifice

- The sacrifice of an evil person is detestable, especially when it is offered with wrong motives.

- Sacrifice is the biggest form of love.

- Obedience is better than sacrifice.

Safety

- Personal liberty ends where public safety begins.

- To avoid trouble and ensure safety, breathe through your nose. It keeps the mouth shut.

- Don't be hasty when it comes to safety.

Satisfaction

- Character grows in the soil of experience, with the fertilization of example, the moisture of desire, and the sunshine of satisfaction.

- It's remarkable how large a part ignorance plays in making a man satisfied with himself.

- Few men are ever satisfied when they get what they deserve.

- Almost anything can be bought at a reduced price except lasting satisfaction.

- Satisfaction is the best kind of internal revenue.

- The greatest reward for serving others is the satisfaction found in your own heart.

- What's the big hurry? You're not ever going to get it done, so what are you racing toward? Every single activity that you're involved in is for one purpose only, and that is to give you a moment of joy. Lighten up. Laugh more. Appreciate more. All is well. – *Abraham-Hicks*

- Wise words satisfy like a good meal; the right words bring satisfaction.

- A person who is full refuses honey, but even bitter food tastes sweet to the hungry.

- I take nothing for granted. I now have only good days and great days.

- People forget how fast you did a job – they remember how well you did it. – *Howard W. Newton*

- Strive to achieve your heart's desires and to release the desires that do not serve you. – *Leon Nacson*

- I feel good praising others so that they feel better about themselves.

- I am content doing work that I love so that the hours' fly.

- It makes me happy to be emotionally self-sufficient although I still enjoy and rejoice in the company and appropriate attention or assistance of others.

SAYINGS

- A word aptly spoken is like apples of gold in settings of silver.

- When you were born, you cried and the world rejoiced. Live your life in such a manner that when you die the world cries and you rejoice. – *Old Indian Saying*

- Common sense is very uncommon. – *Horace Greely*

- Be careful of your thoughts; they may become words at any moment. – *Lara Gassen*

- Experience is what you get when you don't get what you want. – *Dan Stanford*

- I found out that it is not good to talk about my troubles. Eighty percent of people who hear them don't care and the other 20 percent are glad you're having troubles. – *Tommy Lasorda*

SECRETS

- It's a great kindness to entrust people with a secret. They feel so important while telling it to their friends.

- If you want a secret kept — keep it.

- Three people can keep a secret if two of them are dead.

- A secret is usually something that is told to only one person at a time.

- Some folk's idea of keeping a secret is merely refusing to tell who told it to them.

- The only way to keep a secret is not to tell it.

- Secrets are things we give to others to keep for us.

- The secret of success is seldom well-kept.

Self-Control

- He is a fool who cannot get angry, but he is a wise man who will not.

- Never strike a child! You might miss and hurt yourself.

- Striking while the iron is hot may be all right, but don't strike while the head is hot.

- You are not a dynamic person simply because you blow your top.

- Be strong enough to control your anger instead of letting it control you.

- No matter whether you are on the road or in an argument, when you begin to see red, STOP!

- When a person strikes in anger, he usually misses the mark.

- Form the habit of closing your mouth firmly when angry.

- In an argument the best weapon to hold is your tongue.

- We first make our habits, and then our habits make us.

- At no time is self-control more difficult than in time of success.

- Self-expression is good; self-control is better.

- Self-control might be defined as the ability to carry a credit card and not abuse it.

- When a man loses his temper, his reason goes on a vacation.

- It is always a good idea to be selfish with your temper — so always keep it.

Self-Love

- From now on, let every action, every reaction, every thought, and every emotion be based on love. Increase your self-love until the entire dream of your life is transformed from fear and drama to love and joy. – *Don Miguel Ruiz.*

- It is one of the most beautiful compensations of this life that no man can sincerely try to help another without helping himself.

- Love yourself, love your neighbor, love your enemies, but begin with self-love. You cannot love others until you love yourself. You cannot share what you do not have. If you do not love yourself, you cannot love anyone else either. – *Don Miguel Ruiz*

- If you don't love yourself, nobody else will. Not only that — you won't be good at loving anyone else. Loving starts with the self. – *Dr. Wayne W. Dyer*

- Self-love and self-acceptance are the ultimate acts of self-care. – *Cheryl Richardson*

- It is one of the most beautiful compensations of this life that no man can sincerely try to help another without helping himself.

- Have high regard for yourself. Be your own best friend. – *Leon Nacson*

SELFISHNESS

- The person who is all wrapped up in himself is overdressed.

- Some of us veer to the left and some of us swing to the right, but most of us are self-centered.

- A man who is self-centered is off-centered.

- It's give and take in this world, with too many people trying to take.

- Selfishness tarnishes everything it touches.

- He who lives for himself does not have very much to live for.

- The selfish man, like a ball of twine, is wrapped up in himself.

- A man is a selfish fool who says it's nobody's business what he does.

- The trouble with most people is that every time they think, they think only of themselves.

SELF-WORTH

- Acknowledge that you are the source of your manifestations. – *Cherie Carter-Scott Ph.D.*

- It doesn't matter what other people say or do. What matters is how you choose to react and what you choose to believe about yourself. – *Louise L. Hay*

- Once you free your notion of self-worth from the bonds of material things, you will "need" less and you will spend less. As your self-esteem rises, your debt will diminish. Call it a law of financial physics! – *Suze Orman*

SERVICE

- Ask how you can serve the community rather than asking how the community can serve you.

- When you use your calling to make a difference in the community, opportunities to correct.

- Create abundance will emerge in your life. – *Tavis Smiley*

- The end depends on the beginning; public service is a noble calling. A life of service must include serving others.

- Contribute to others through your work, your friendships, and through anonymous service. Your concern need only be blessing the lives of others. Influence, not recognition, becomes the true motive. – *Stephen R. Covey*

SIGHT

- What we see is mainly what we look for.

- Seeing is believing.

- There are none so blind as those who have eyes but will not see.

- The only thing worse than being blind is having sight but no vision.

Silence

- You must speak up to be heard, but sometimes you have to shut up to be appreciated.

- When an argument flares up, the wise man quenches it with silence.

- The secret of polite conversation is never to open your mouth unless you have something to say.

- A wise man reflects before he speaks; a fool speaks and then reflects on what he has uttered.

- Never neglect the opportunity of keeping your mouth shut.

- Speech is silver, silence is golden, and oratory, at the moment, is mainly brass.

- Try to understand silence — it's worth listening to.

- If silence is golden, not many people can be arrested for hoarding.

- Silence never makes any blunders.

- The best way to say a thing is to say it, unless remaining silent will say it better.

- Silence is often the most perfect expression of scorn.

- Most of us know how to say nothing, but few of us know when.

- You can learn a lot about a man by how much he doesn't say.

- Very seldom can you improve on saying nothing.

- People who can hold their tongues rarely have any trouble holding their friends.

- Wise men are not always silent, but they know when to be.

- If you don't say it, you won't have to unsay it.

- Let's keep our mouths shut and our pens dry until we know the facts.

- Silence is at its golden best when you keep it long enough to get all the facts.

- Truth is often violated by falsehood, but can be equally outraged by silence.

Sincerity

- Be sincere with your compliments. Most people can tell the difference between sugar and saccharine.

- The sincere man suspects that he, too, is sometimes guilty of the faults he sees in others.

- A fellow ought to be sincere whether he means it or not!

- The sincerity of a person does not make false doctrine right just because he believes it.

- Be open, honest, and honorable in all your endeavors. Establish high standards, principles and values for yourself, then kick up a level. In everything you do, be true to yourself. – *Tavis Smiley*

- As a face is reflected in water, so the heart reflects the real person.

- In the end, people appreciate honest criticism far more than flattery.

- Wounds from a sincere friend are better than many kisses from an enemy.

- The heartfelt counsel of a friend is as sweet as perfume and incense.

- Don't count the days, make the days count. – *Muhammad Ali*

- It's better to speak from your heart with everyone you communicate with. Otherwise, anger will creep in, and you'll resent the person or the obligation. – *Brian L. Weiss, M.D.*

- When we give it our all, we can live with ourselves regardless of results.

- Decide what your highest priorities are, and have the courage and independent willpower to say no- pleasantly, smilingly, and unapologetically- to the things that are less important to you. – *Stephen R. Covey*

Solitude

- Cultivate a loving relationship with yourself. Be willing to be alone and enjoy your own company. – *Christian Northrup, M.D.*

- Some people see things as they are and say why. I see things as they never were and say why not.

- Make time to relax, be still, and enjoy your solitude, indulging in much-needed self-care. – *Doreen Virtue, Ph.D.*

Speech

- The recipe for a good speech includes quite a bit of shortening.

- A good speech is one with a good beginning and a good ending, which are kept very close together.

- A speech should be like a woman's skirt — long enough to cover the subject, but short enough to be interesting.

- Wisdom is knowing when to speak your mind and when to mind your speech.

- Out of the abundance of the heart, the mouth speaketh.

SPOUSE

- A man scores points with a woman if he does his best to contribute. A woman scores points with a man when she lets him off the hook when he makes a mistake. – *John Gray*

- Men, think out your thoughts before you express anger toward her. Women, use soft language when you express your anger toward him. – *John Gray*

- When a woman is overwhelmed, she retreats to her "well" to recharge. When man becomes angry, he needs to go to his "cave" to cool off. – *John Gray*

- She values love, communication, beauty, and relationships. He appreciates admiration, recognition and trust. – *John Gray*

- The more a woman feels the right to be upset, the less upset she will be. When men talk about their problems, they're looking for solutions. *– John Gray*

- Women do not appreciate being told how to change their feelings. Men do not like being told what to do. *– John Gray*

- Women love to care for their men, but primarily, they need to feel cared for themselves. Men need to feel cared, but primarily, they need to feel successful in fulfilling their partners. *– John Gray*

- Men have sight, women have insight.

- Women thrive on communication because it nurtures their female side. Men thrive on appreciation because it nurtures their male side. *– John Gray*

- A woman expects her partner to know when she needs support. A man asks for support when he needs it. *– John Gray*

- A man's greatest challenge is to take responsibility for his contribution to a problem. A woman's greatest challenge is to let go of her resentment and find forgiveness. – *John Gray*

❦ Man, think out your thoughts before you express anger toward her. Woman, use soft language when you express your anger toward him. – *John Gary*

❦ Women put everyone else first. If we put women first, we put ourselves, first. – *Tony Elumelu*

Steadfastness

❦ Say yes until you believe it.

❦ Stand up for what you believe in.

❦ Stay as constant as the north star.

Stinginess

❦ Beware of a Christian with an open mouth and a closed pocketbook.

- Generosity will always leave a more pleasant memory then stinginess.

- Some folks give according to their means, and some give according to their meanness.

- Many people are not exactly stingy — they're just economical in a very obnoxious way.

- The only time a miser puts his hand in his pocket is during cold weather.

STRENGTH

- Be strong enough to control your anger instead of letting it control you.

- The strength that comes from confidence can be quickly lost in conceit.

- Greatness lies not in being strong, but in the right use of strength.

- Weak men wait for opportunities; strong men make them.

- Strength in prayer is better than length in prayer.

A SELECTION OF WORDS OF WISDOM AND AFFIRMATIONS FOR MEANINGFUL LIVING AND HAPPINESS

- Trouble is what gives a fellow a chance to discover his strength — or lack of it.

- The weakness of man is the thing to be feared, not his strength.

- Don't ask for an easier life, ask for a stronger person.

- Nothing is so strong as gentleness, nothing is so gentle as real strength.

- You must not only aim right but draw the bow with all your might. – *Henry David Thoreau*

- Don't ask for an easier life, ask to be a stronger person.

- Strength does not come from physical capacity. It comes from an indomitable will. – *Mahatma Ghandi*

- Strength is nothing more than enduring life—to be able to survive the heartaches and agonies we go through with our heads held high. Sometimes just walking through adversity to get to the other side is a sign of strength. – *Sylvia Browne*

Success

- Winners never quit. Quitters never win. The man who gets ahead is the man who does more than is necessary — and keeps on doing it.

- Successful men follow the same advice they prescribe for others.

- If you want to go far in business, you'll have to stay close to it.

- Enthusiasm is the propelling force necessary for climbing the ladder of success.

- There are two elements of success: aspiration and perspiration.

- If at first you don't succeed, try try again.

- For success, try aspiration, inspiration, and perspiration.

- Formula for success: When you start a thing, finish it.

- Success is sweet, but its secret is sweat.

- No one has yet climbed the ladder of success with his hands in his pockets.

- Some men succeed by what they know, some by what they do, and a few by what they are.

- The secret of success and happiness lies not in doing what you like, but in liking what you do.

- One secret of success is to be able to put your best foot forward without stepping on anybody's toes.

- One thing that keeps a lot of people from being a success is work.

- Success is journey, not a destination.

- Success is not something to wait for; it is something you work for. – *ASU Psychology and Dept. of Education Bulletin*

- The 5 F's of success; focus, finish, follow up, follow through, and faith.

- The price of success is perseverance. The price of failure comes cheaper.

- When a woman succeeds, the family succeeds, the community succeeds and the continent succeeds. – *Tony Elumelu*

SUSPICION

- Suspicion is like a pair of dark glasses — it makes all the world look dark.

- Most of our suspicion of others is aroused by a knowledge of ourselves.

- The easiest thing in the world to cultivate is suspicion.

- Suspicion is a mental picture seen through an imaginary keyhole.

SYMPATHY

- Children need strength to lean on, a shoulder to cry on, and an example to learn from.

- Friendship is a living thing that lasts only as long as it is nourished with kindness, sympathy, and understanding.

- The true measure of a man is the height of his ideals, the breadth of his sympathy, the depth of his convictions, and the length of his patience.

- A person who is not sympathetic is simply pathetic.

- Sympathy is the result of thinking with your heart.

- The only time sympathy is ever wasted is when you give it to yourself.

- One manifestation of genuine sympathy is worth more than any amount of advice.

- Sympathy is the golden key that unlocks the hearts of others.

- Be sympathetic — you know it could happen to you!

- Rejoice with them that do rejoice. And weep with them that weep.

- Sympathy is your pain in my heart. – *Halford E. Luccock*

- Who would recognize the unhappy if grief had no language? – *Publilius Syrus*

- There is no greater loan then a sympathetic ear. – *Frank Tyger*

- Anyone can sympathize with the sufferings of a friend, but it requires a very fine nature to sympathize with a friend's success. – *Oscar Wilde*

- Sympathy is you're in my heart. – *Halford E. Luccock*

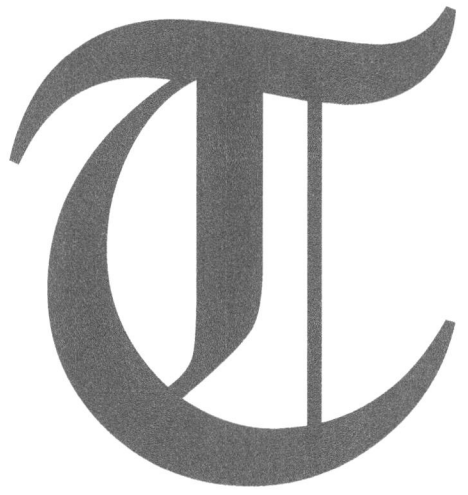

TACT

- The real art of conversation is not only saying the right thing in the right place, but to leave unsaid the wrong thing at the tempting moment.

- People with tact have less to retract.

- Tact is the rare talent for not quite telling the truth.

- Tact is the ability to describe others as they see themselves.

- Tact is the ability not to say what you really think.

- Tact is the art of saying whatever is required — including nothing.

- Making people around you think they know something is real tact.

- Some people have tact, others tell the truth.

- Tact is the ability to stay in the middle of the road without being caught there.

- Formula for tact: Be brief, politely; be aggressive, smilingly; be emphatic, pleasantly; be positive, diplomatically; be right, graciously.

- Tact is the knack of getting your way without stirring up a fuss.

- Tact fails the moment it is noticed.

- Tact is the art of saying nothing when there is nothing to say.

- Tact is the unsaid part of what you think.

- Blunt words often have the sharpest edge.

TEACHING

- Education's purpose is to replace an empty mind with an open one. – *Malcom S. Forbes*

- The mediocre teacher tells, the good teacher explains, the superior teacher demonstrates The great teacher inspires. – *William Arthur Ward*

- To teach is to learn. – *Japanese Proverb*

- The teacher who is attempting to teach without inspiring the pupil with a desire to learn is hammering on cold iron. – *Horac Mann*

- We are all students and teachers. Ask yourself: *"What did I come here to learn, and what did I come here to teach?" – Louise L. Hay*

Temper

- The world needs more warm hearts and fewer hot heads.

- People who fly into a rage always make a bad landing.

- Some people think they have dynamic personalities because they're always exploding.

- Temper gets people into trouble, but pride keeps them there.

- If you lose your head, how do you expect to be able to use it?

- When you're right you can afford to keep your temper; when you're wrong you can't afford to lose it.

- You'll never get to the top if you keep blowing yours.

- The most important time to hold your temper is when the other person has lost his.

- Striking while the iron is hot is all right, but don't strike while the head is hot.

- When a man loses his temper, his reason goes on a vacation.

- A temper displayed in public is indecent exposure.

- It is always a good idea to be selfish with your temper — so always keep it.

- It is extremely difficult for a man who loses his temper to hold his friends.

- Keep your temper. Nobody else wants it.

- Keep your temper to yourself. It's useless to others.

- When your temper boils over, you are usually in hot water.

Temptation

- You'll make a huge spiritual leap forward when you begin to focus less on beating temptation and more on avoiding it. – *Dr. Bruce Wilkinson*

- Better shun the bait than struggle in the snare. – *J. Hudson Taylor*

- The trouble with opportunity is that it only knocks. Temptation kicks the door in. – *Anonymous*

Testimony

- Truth has no special time of its own. Its hour is now — always. – *Albert Schweitzer*

- One man practicing sportsmanship is far better than 50 preaching it. – *Knute Rockne*

- A good sermon helps people in two ways. Some rise from it greatly strengthened, others wake from it refreshed. – *E.C mckenzie*

Thankfulness

- Thankfulness could well be the finest sentiment of man — and also the rarest.

- If you have nothing for which to be thankful, make up your mind that there's something wrong with you.

- We should be thankful for the good things that we have and, also, for the bad things we don't have.

Thoughts

- Kind actions begin with kind thoughts.

- Do it now! Today will be yesterday tomorrow.

- The actions of men are the best interpreters of their thoughts.

- Language is the dress of thought; every time you talk your mind is on parade.

- People with a one — track mind often have a derailed train of thought.

- The one thing worse than a vacant mind is one filled with spiteful thoughts.

- Be careful of your thoughts. They may break out into words at any time.

- He is never alone who is in the company of noble thoughts.

- See that you have a supply of worthy thoughts before you begin to talk.

- You cannot escape the results of your own thoughts.

- Human thought is like a pendulum — it keeps swinging from one extreme to another.

- Our words may hide our thoughts, but our actions will reveal them.

- Positive thinking will let you do everything better than negative thinking will. – *Zig Ziglar*

- Two reasonable heads are better than one.

- Good thoughts bear good fruits. Bad thoughts bear bad fruits. A man is his own gardener. – *James Allen*

Treasure

- Search for them as you would for silver; seek them like hidden treasures.

- There is treasure in the house of the godly, but the earnings of the wicked bring trouble.

- The greatest treasures are those invisible to the eye but found by the heart.

- One man's clutter; is another man's treasure.

Treatment

- A single rebuke does more for a person of understanding than a hundred lashes on the back of a fool.

- How you treat people — whether it be an old friend or a teller at the bank — is indicative of how you can expect people to treat you. – *Deepak Chopra, M.D.*

- Do unto others as you would have them do unto you.

- One good turn deserves another.

Thrift

- In the "good old days" the man who saved money was a miser. Now he's a wonder.

- Try to save money. Someday it may be valuable again.

- It's easier to admire the other fellow's thrift than to practice it yourself.

- Wisdom enables one to be thrifty without being stingy, and generous without being wasteful.

- What Mother Nature giveth, Father Time taketh away.

- No wonder time flies. Have you ever noticed how many people are out to kill it?

- Killing time is not murder, it's suicide.

- When you kill time, just remember it has no resurrection.

- Time is what we want the most, and what we use the worst.

- The busy man seems to have time for everything. The man who just thinks he's busy hasn't time for anything.

- Whenever we waste time, we should remember that Father Time never makes a round trip.

- Hours and flowers soon fade away.

- Time is like money — you can only spend it once.

- Lost time is never found again.

- Time can be wasted but never recycled.

- The only person who saves time is the one who spends it wisely.

TROUBLE

- A troublemaker plants seeds of strife; gossip separates the best of friends.

- Those who bring trouble on their families inherit the wind. The fool will be a servant to the wise.

- A person who plans evil will get a reputation as a troublemaker.

- Real friendship is shown in times of trouble; prosperity is full of friends.

TIME

- No hand can make the clock strike for me the hours that are passed. – *George Gordon Byron*

- Time and tide wait for no man. – *Geoffrey Chaucer*

- Time is too slow for those who wait, too swift for those who fear, too long for those who grieve, too short for those who rejoice, but for those who love, time is eternity. – *Henry Van Dyke*

- Time is what we want most, but what we use worst.

TOLERANCE

- The chief evil of many people consists not so much in doing evil, but in permitting it.

- Good manners are being able to put up with bad ones.

- An open mind tolerates an empty one.

- Tolerance is seeing things with your heart instead of your eyes.

- It is extremely difficult for the tolerant to tolerate the intolerant.

- Tolerance starts when you practice it, not when you just talk about it.

- Tolerance often gets the credit that belongs to indifference.

- Tolerance is the patience shown by a wise man when he listens to an ignoramus.

TRUST

- Allow and empower someone you trust to guide you on your path. – *Cherie Carter-Scott, Ph.D.*

- When life presents more challenges than you can handle, delegate to God. He not only has the answer, He is the answer. – *Tavis Smiley*

- Trust is the essence of win-win relationships. Because you trust others and they trust you, you can be open; you can put your cards on the table. Even though you may see things differently, you're committed to understanding each other's viewpoints. – *Stephen R. Covey*

- Trust takes years to build, seconds to break, and forever to repair.

- A gossip goes around telling secrets, but those who are trustworthy can keep a confidence.

- Trustworthy messengers refresh like snow in the summer. They revive the spirit of their employer.

TRUTH

- There's nothing so kingly as kindness, and nothing so royal as truth.

- The truth may hurt but a lie is agony.

- Truth often hurts, but it's the lie that leaves the scars.
- Some people have tact, others tell the truth.
- Nothing is harder for some folks to see than the naked truth.
- The surest way to be lonesome is to always tell the truth.
- Truth never dies, but it is often paralyzed by man's indifference.
- When truth stands in your way, it's time to change directions.
- The greatest homage you can pay the truth is to use it.
- The truth is one thing for which there are no known substitutes.
- Truth fears nothing but concealment.
- Truth is something which must be known with the mind, accepted with the heart, and enacted in life.
- To hear truth and not accept it does not nullify it.
- Truth is so stubborn it doesn't apologize to anybody.

- Truth angers those whom it does not fully convince.

- Truth is not always popular, but is always right.

- Say the truth and it will make you free.

- The truth hurts — especially when someone's telling it about you.

- Words sometimes serve as a smoke screen to obscure the truth, rather than as a searchlight to reveal it.

- Truthful words stand the test of time, but lies are soon exposed.

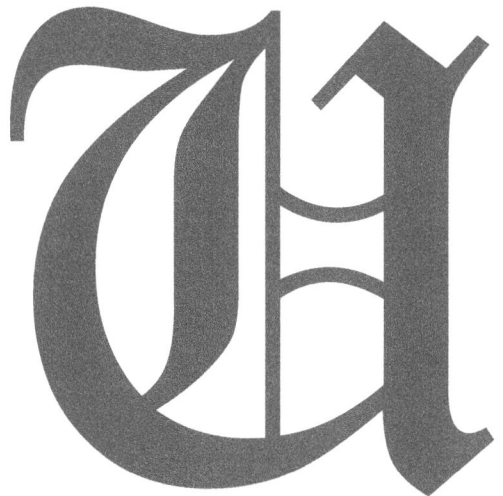

Understanding

- The wise are known for their understanding, and pleasant words are persuasive.

- We are all unique. Understand rather than judge.

- What the mind doesn't understand, it worships or fears.

- Cry out for insight, and ask for understanding.

Unity

- When we are unified, working together, no challenge is insurmountable. – *Paul Kagame*

- United we stand, divided we fall. – *John Dickinson*

- Humility will lead us to unity, and unity will lead to peace.

- I can do things you cannot. You can do things I cannot. Together, we can do great things.

UNIQUE

- I am wonderful and unique because I am the only "me" in the world.

- I respect the uniqueness of all others and I will try to understand each person I meet or know rather than always see them through my own history or perceptions.

- Always have a unique character like salt, its presence is felt but its absence makes everything tasteless.

- In order to be irreplaceable one must always be different.

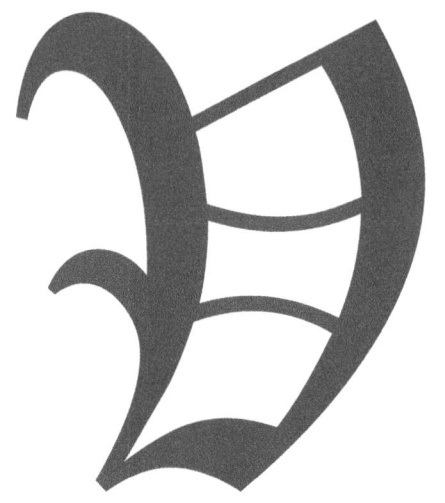

VALUES

- It is extremely easy for us to give our major attention to minor matters.

- Be slow in choosing friends, slower in changing them.

- The things in life that count most are the things that can't be counted.

- A little pride is a small thing to lose when compared with losing honor.

- In your search for riches, don't lose the things that money can't buy.

- The relative value of health and wealth depends on which you have left.

- The highest values are priceless.

- Some things cannot be measured. We do not think of a ton of truth, a bushel of beauty, or an inspiration a mile long.

- The value of all things, even our lives, depends on the use we make of them.

- People who talk about things they can't afford sometimes forget that the list should include pride, envy, and malice.

- The things of greatest value in life are those things that multiply when divided.

- A sense of value is the most important single element in human personality.

- Spiritual bankruptcy is inevitable when a man is no longer able to keep the interest paid on his moral obligations.

- It is what we value, not what we have, that makes us rich.

- Try not to become a person of success but rather try to become a person of value. – *Albert Einstein*

Verbosity

- Words are like leaves. Where they most abound, the fruit of sense beneath is rarely found.

- Verbosity is the enemy of eloquence.

- Verbosity leads to unclear, inarticulate things.

VICES

- Vices are to be condemned and eradicated, not condoned and taxed for revenue.

- Man's greatest vices are the misuses of his virtues.

- Cultivate vices when you are young, and when you are old they will not forsake you.

- Virtues are usually learned at mother's knee, and vices are learned at some other joint.

VICTORY

- Accept the challenges, so that you may feel the exhilaration of victory.

- Victory belongs to the most persevering.

- The harder the battle, the sweeter the victory.

Virtue

- Sometimes we learn more from a man's errors than from his virtues.

- A fault which humbles a man is of more use to him than a virtue which puffs him up.

- Gratitude is the rarest of all virtues, and yet we invariably expect it.

- The path of the virtuous leads away from evil; whoever follows that path is safe.

- The virtue lies in the struggle, not in the prize.

- Gratitude is not only the greatest of virtues, but the parent of all the others.

- We all agree that the nicest people in the world are those who minimize our faults and magnify our virtues.

- Sometimes virtue and prosperity have trouble living together.

- To know what not to think about is a major intellectual virtue.

- When one robs another of virtue, he loses his own.

- Virtues are usually learned at mother's knee, and vices are learned at some other joint.

- If our good deeds were immediately and invariably rewarded, then virtue would become a racket.

- Virtue has more admirers than followers.

- Some identify happiness with good fortune, though others identify it with virtue.

Vision

- Conceit is a form of "I" strain that doctors can't cure.

- Faith is the daring of the soul to go farther than it can see.

- Few people have good enough sight to see their own faults.

- We usually see things, not as they are, but as we are.

- If it is not fit to live in, then our job is to make it fit.
  – *Fela Kuti*

❦ The very essence of leadership is that you have to have a vision. You can't blow an uncertain trumpet. – *Jonathan Swift*

❦ Begin today with the image of the end of your life as your frame of reference by which everything else is examined. Each day will then contribute to the vision you have of your life as a whole. – *Stephen R. Covey*

VOCATION

❦ Choose a job you love and you will never have to work a day in your life. – *Confucius*

❦ Work spares us from three great evils: boredom, vice and need. – *Voltaire*

❦ Don't tell me how hard you work. Tell me how much you get done. – *James Ling*

❦ People who make a living doing something they don't enjoy wouldn't even be happy with a one-day work week. – *Edward "Duke" Ellington*

❦ The person who knows "how" will always have a job. The person who knows "why" will always be his boss. — *Diane Ravitch*

❦ Uneasy lies the head that wears a crown. — *Benjamin Franklin*

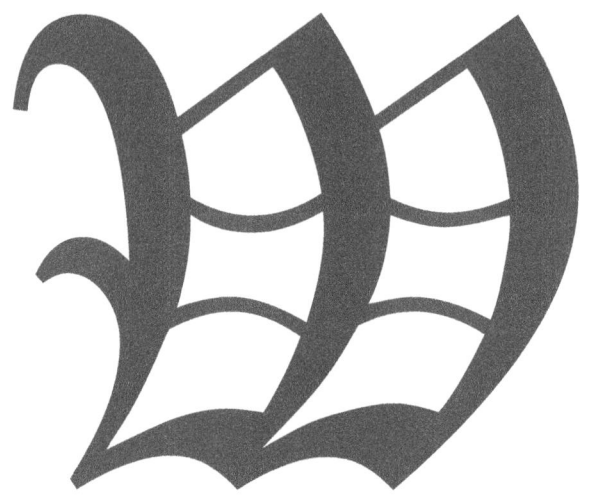

WAR

- The drums of war are easy to beat but the rhythms are difficult to dance. – *Ibrahim Babangida*

- He who fights and runs will live to fight another day.

- If wars can be started by lies, they can be stopped by truth.

WEAKNESS

- To be angry with a weak man is proof that you are not very strong yourself.

- The weakness of man is the thing to be feared, not his strength.

- Weak men wait for opportunities; strong men make them.

- Profanity is the use of strong words by weak people.

Wealth

- It is not by a man's purse, but by his character, that he is rich or poor.

- Men of genius are admired; men of wealth are envied; men of power are feared; but only men of character are trusted.

- The rich think of their wealth as a strong defense; they imagine it to be a high wall of safety.

- When disaster strikes, you won't have to ask your brother for assistance.

- The greatest wealth is contentment with a little.

- Contentment in life consists not in great wealth, but in simple wants.

- A lot of people lose their health trying to become wealthy, and then lose their wealth trying to get back their health.

- Those who ignore health in the pursuit of wealth usually wind up losing both.

- It is not wealth, but the arrogance of wealth, that offends the poor.

- There are two ways to become wealthy: spend less and earn more.

Wickedness

- The wicked are punished in place of the godly, and traitors in place of the honest.

- When the wicked take charge, people go into hiding. When the wicked meet disaster the godly flourish.

- The godly will never be disturbed, but the wicked will be removed from the land.

- There is no rest for the wicked until we close our eyes for good.

Will

- Nothing is difficult to those who have will.

- The difference between a successful person and others is not a lack of strength, not a lack of knowledge, but rather in a lack of will. – *Vincent T. Lombardi*

- Strength does not come from physical capacity. It comes from an indomitable will. – *Mahatma Gandhi*

- Where there is a will, there is a way.

WISDOM

- Advice is that which the wise don't need and fools won't take.

- Years make all of us old and very few of us wise.

- Joyful is the person who finds wisdom, the one who gains understanding.

- Fools think their own way is right, but the wise listen to others.

- Wise people think before they act; fools don't and even brag about their foolishness.

- Some people make cutting remarks, but the words of the wise bring healing.

- Walk with the wise and become wise; associate with fools and get in trouble.

- The wise don't make a show of their knowledge, but fools broadcast their foolishness.

- The age of Methuselah has nothing to do with the wisdom of Solomon.

- Wise people sometimes change their minds — fools, never.

- Knowledge comes by taking things apart, but wisdom comes by putting things together.

- Knowledge is knowing a fact. Wisdom is knowing what to do with that fact.

- Wise men are not always silent, but they know when to be.

- To know what to do with what you know is the essence of wisdom.

- Wise men always know more than they tell, but fools tell more than they know.

- Wisdom is knowing when to speak your mind and when to mind your speech.

- Wisdom is knowledge in action.

- The wise man uses his mouth less, eyes more, ears more — and knows more.

WORDS

- It is always best to keep your words soft and sweet, you might never know when you'd have to eat them.
  – Ola Rotimi

- Action speaks louder than words — and speak fewer lies.

- People may doubt what you say, but they will always believe what you do.

- Superior to a kind thought is a kind word; better than both is a kind deed.

- The soundness of your ideas is more important than the sound of your words.

- A lot of indigestion is caused by people having to eat their own words.

- Let all your words be kind, and you will always hear kind echoes.

- Works, not words, are the proof of love.

- Beware of using sharp words. You may have to eat them later on down the line.

- The written word can be erased — not so with the spoken word.

- Kind words are short to speak, but their echoes are endless.

- Blunt words often have the sharpest edge.

- Kind words do not wear out the tongue — so speak them.

- Words can make a deeper scar than silence can ever heal.

- It is vain to use words when deeds are expected.

- Words and feathers are easily scattered, but not easily gathered up.

- A spoken word and a thrown stone cannot be recalled.

- The man of few words doesn't have to take many of them back.

- In the use of words, quality is more important than quantity.

- Our words may hide our thoughts, but our actions will reveal them.

WORTH

- The highest reward for a person's toil is not what they get for it, but what they become by it.

- No one can depress you. No one can make you anxious. No one can hurt your feelings. No one can make you anything other than what you allow inside. – *Dr. Wayne W. Dyer*

- For better or worse, you're responsible for everything your past and future. Don't blame your parents, your teachers, or your boss. Take it on yourself. – *Tavis Smiley*

- Never look down on anybody unless you're helping him up. – *Jesse Jackson*

- The house of the wicked will be destroyed, but the tent of the godly will flourish.

WORK

- Some fellows dream of worthy accomplishments, while others stay awake and do them.

- Ambition never gets anywhere until it forms a partnership with work.

- If you want to go far in business, you'll have to stay close to it.

- A man has happiness in the palm of his hands if he can fill his days with real work and his nights with real rest.

- A task worth doing and friends worth having make life worthwhile.

- Nothing worthwhile is achieved without patience, labor, and disappointment.

- Success is sweet, but its secret is sweat.

- Most people do only what they are required to do, but successful people do a little more.

- Unless we all work for the common good there won't be any.

- It is better to become bent from hard work than to become crooked without it.

- Hard work never hurts people who don't do any.

- Two things deprive people of their peace of mind: work unfinished, and work not yet begun.

- Hard work rarely kills because so few give it a chance.

- One of the hardest ways to make a living is to work for it.

- A man's work is a portrait of himself.

- The young man who is able to work his way through college is a pretty good bet to be able to work his way through life.

- Dodging work is the hardest work of all and yields the poorest returns.

- The best way to criticize the other fellow's work is to do yours better.

- If hard work is the key to success, most people would rather pick the lock.

- The reason worry kills more people than work is that people worry more than they work.

WORRY

- There will always be enough for today without taking on yesterday and tomorrow's burdens.

- An educated man will sit up all night and worry over things a fool never dreamed of.

- Every tomorrow has two handles. We can take hold of it by the handle of anxiety, or by the handle of faith.

- A lot of people who are worrying about the future ought to be preparing for it.

- More people worry about the future than prepare for it.

- If you live within your income, you'll live without worry — and without a lot of other things.

- The best way to live a long life is to get somebody to do the worrying for you.

- The greatest mistake you can make in this life is to be constantly fearful you will make one.

- Instead of counting their blessings many people magnify their problems.

- Worry weighs a person down; an encouraging word cheers a person up.

- Never worry about the tide that is going out. It always comes back.

- Worry can't change the past, but it can ruin the present.

- Those who live in a worry invite death in a hurry.

- Worry never changes a single thing — except the worrier.

- Worry never accomplishes anything except wrinkles — which gives you another thing to worry about.

- One good rule for living is not to worry about the future until we have learned to manage the present.

- The reason worry kills more people than work is that people worry more than they work.

- To worry about what we can't help is useless; to worry about what we can help is stupid.

- Don't worry too much about what lies ahead. Go as far as you can see, and when you get there, you can see farther.

- Worry often gives a small thing a big shadow.

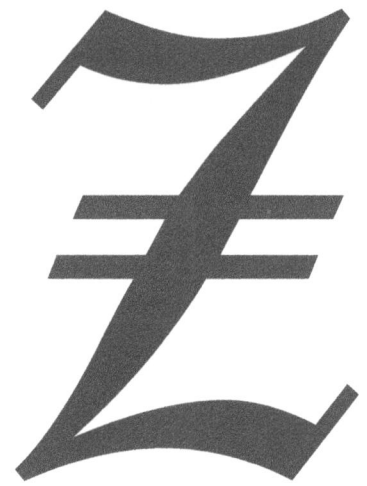

ZEAL

- There's always a good crop of food for thought. What we need is enough enthusiasm to harvest it.

- He who has no fire in himself cannot warm others.

- Zeal without knowledge is like heat without light.

- There is no zeal so intemperate and cruel as that which is backed by ignorance.

- Zeal without knowledge is the sister of folly.

- Young entrepreneurs and those they inspire are the lifeblood of Africa's rise. – *Tony Elumelu*

Prayer/Song Affirmations

For Protection

* I am made in the image and likeness of Christ and nothing harmful shall happen to me. I am protected.
*Protect me according to thy goodwill and pleasure from violent sudden and unnatural death and from all other evil accidents for thou at my help and my God and thine is the power and glory, Amen Selah

For Repentance

*Jesus Lord, I ask for mercy; let me not implore in vain, all my sins I now detest them. Never will I sin again

For Interviews

*El Eyon, most strong and highest God, may it please thee to change the heart of my enemies and opposers that they may do me good instead of evil as thou didst in the days of Abraham when he Called upon thee by this holy name, Amen Selah.

For Examination

O Virgin Mother, lady of good counsel sweetest picture artists ever drew. In all my doubts, I fly to thee for guidance. O mother tell me what I am to do.
Trust and Obey for there is no other way to be happy in Jesus but to trust and obey.

For Guidance/Protection

O may this bounteous God, through
all our life be near us. With ever
joyful hearts, And blesses peace to
cheer us; And keep us in his grace, And
guide us when perplexed, And
free us from all ills, In this world
and the next.

*Those contributed by Dr. Acholonu's father, Willfred W. Acholonu

For Guidance

It's not an easy road, we are
travelling to heaven. For many are
the thorns on the way. It's not an easy road

but the Saviour is with us; His presence gives us joy every day.

For Thanksgiving

My soul now glorify, the Lord who is
my Saviour, Rejoice for whom am I
That God has shown me favour?

For Protection

I need thee every hour
Most precious Lord
No tender voice like thine
Can peace afford.

For Blessing

I need thee, Oh I need thee,
Every hour I need thee
Oh, bless me now, my saviour
I come to see thee.

For Help

I need thee every hour

In joy or pain
Come quickly and abide
Or life is vain.
I need thee every hour
Most Holy One
Oh, make me thine indeed
thou blessed son.

For Mercy and Compassion

God of mercy and compassion
Look with pity upon me;
Father, let me call thee Father
As thy child returns to thee.

For Trust

On Christ the solid rock I stand
All other ground is sinking sand
All other ground is sinking sand.

For Hope

When darkness seems to hide his
face, I rest on his unchanging grace
In every high and stormy gale

My anchor holds within the vale.

Jesus my Saviour is all things to me
Oh what a wonderful Saviour is He
Guiding protection o'er life's
troubled sea
Mighty deliver Jesus form.

For Help

O God, our help in ages past,
Our hope for years to come,
Our shelter from the stormy blast
And our eternal home.

O God, our help in ages past
Our hope for years to come
Be thou our guard while troubles
 last; And our eternal home.

O Queen of the Rosemary hail
Immaculate Mother of grace
O pray for us, help us today
Thou hope of the human race.

REFERENCES

Great Quotations, Publishing company 1997. Teacher's inspirations, Great Quotations, Inc. Glendale HTS, IL pp 77

Hay, Louise. L and Friends 2004. Everyday positive thinking. Hay House, Inc. Carlsbad CA. pp 445

Hughey, B & J. 1994. A rainbow of hope. Rainbow studies, Inc. El Reno, OKC pp 336

McKenzie, E. C. Year? 14,000 Quips & Quotes for writers & speakers. Crown Publishers, Inc. NY pp 581

Wilson, G. M. 2013. Words of wisdom. Tyndale House Publishers, Inc. Carol Stream, Illinois

Yager, J. 2011. 365 daily affirmations for happiness. Hannacroix Creek Books, Inc. Stamford, Connecticut pp 107.

International Airport, Lagos, Nigeria 2020. Words of wisdom from International Airport

Willy-Esther Foundation Calendar 2014

Willy-Esther Foundation Calendar 2018 Motivation

Willy-Esther Foundation Calendar 2020

Willy-Esther Foundation Calendar 2021

About The Author

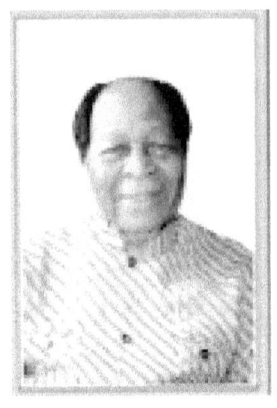

Dr. Alex D. Wozuzu Acholonu has been an emeritus professor of biology at Alcorn State University since 2018 when he retired. He has a Ph.D. degree from Colorado State University (1964) and has expertise in parasitology, microbiology, and environmental biology. He has a certificate in public health and tropical medicine from Tulane University, New Orleans, Louisiana (1994). He was an academic administrator who held all positions in academia — Departmental Chair, Dean of Liberal Studies, Rector (President) of the College of Technology, and Pro-Chancellor (higher than a Vice-chancellor).

He is a nationally and internationally recognized educator who has published three books including, *"Medical Laboratory Diagnosis: Collection, Handling and Storage of Pathological Specimens for Laboratory Investigation"*, his autobiography, *"My Journey Through Life"* and his third one, *"A Selection of Words of Wisdom and Affirmations for Meaningful Living and Happiness"*, two booklets, four book chapters, and more than one hundred and eleven publications as well as many magazine and newspaper articles. He has excelled in his field of expertise and has won many national and international recognitions and accolades. He is cited as one of the 2000 outstanding intellectuals of the 21st century, as one of the great minds of the 21st century by the International Biographical Center, Cambridge, England. He received a universal award for accomplishments in microbiology and parasitology from the American Biographical Institute, one of the top 100 educators of the year (2005), and Who's Who among America's Teachers (2004-2005). He is a recipient of the Nigerian National Honors Award (Medal) of Officer of the Order of the Niger (OON) in 2003 given to him by the then President of Nigeria in recognition of his accomplishments.

He is a recipient of the Mississippi Academy of Science award of Distinguished Contribution to Science and Healthcare Disparity award. He has several fellowships which include a Fellow of the Nigerian Society for parasitology (FNSP), a Fellow of the Renewable and Alternative Energy Society (FRAES), a Fellow of the Mississippi Academy of Science (FMAS), and a Fellow of the Nigerian Academy of Science (FAS), (the highest honor given to a scientist in Nigeria). He was an Executive Board member of the World Federation of Parasitologists (1998 to 2006). He was the chairman of the Division of

Zoology and Entomology of the Mississippi Academy of Sciences several times and chair of the healthcare disparity committee (2016 to 2021). He served as President of the Faculty Senate of Alcorn State University in Mississippi from 1999 to 2004. He is currently the editor-in-chief of Advances in Science and Technologies Journal, (2007 to date) and Community Voice Action Magazine (2016 to date). Dr. Acholonu has been very active in research which took him to many parts of the world (51 countries).

He was one of those selected to participate in the 2005 academic scholars' program in China as a visiting scholar to teach at Huaiyin Teacher's University from May 20th to June 5th, 2005. He has supervised the research of many undergraduate and graduate students. In 2002, he was appointed a member of the Food Advisory Committee of the US Food and Drug Administration (FDA) to serve in this capacity from 2002 to 2005 because of his expertise in microbiology and parasitology and received a distinguished service award in 2005 from FDA. He served as chairman of a review panel of the US Department of Agriculture, in 2016. One of his most outstanding research accomplishments is his discovery, naming, and description of 14 new species of parasites. He served as coordinator of Research Training and Education, Center of Excellence in minority health and health disparity (NIH/NIMHD),

School of Public Health, Jackson State University, Jackson, Mississippi from 2010 to 2018. Dr. Acholonu was married to Lolo Mary Ekeoma Acholonu (now late). They have 7 grown-up children and 16 grandchildren.

www.ingramcontent.com/pod-product-compliance
Lightning Source LLC
Chambersburg PA
CBHW041125110526
44592CB00020B/2686